NEW NORMALS

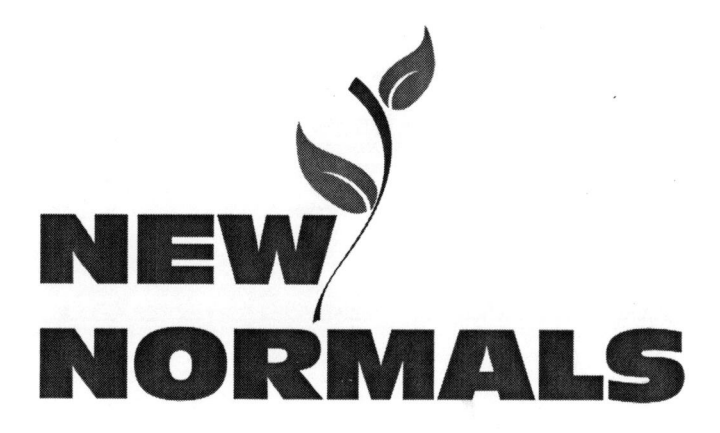

Reclaiming a Life of Significance

A Guide
for Caregivers,
Survivors &
Families of
Stroke/Brain Injury

PAM PAPAS

NEW NORMALS
Reclaiming a Life of Significance

Copyright © 2009 by Pamela A. Papas

All rights reserved. No part of this publication can be reproduced, stored in a retrieval system or photocopied, recorded or otherwise without prior written permission of the publisher.

ISBN 978-0-9819755-0-4

Papas Press LLC
PO BOX 935
Hanover, PA. 17331
www.papaspress.com

Cover design by: Kimberly Martin, www.self-pub.net

Disclaimer

This is not a medical book. It is not intended to replace the advice of your doctor. The information provided in this book should not be construed as personal medical advice or instruction. No action should be taken based solely on the contents of this book. Readers should consult appropriate health professionals on any matter relating to their health and well being. The information and opinions provided here are believed to be accurate and sound, based on the best judgment available to the author, but readers who fail to consult appropriate health authorities assume the risk of any injuries. This book is not responsible for errors or omissions. Before you attempt any exercise routine or therapy it should be preapproved by your doctor or therapist. Each stroke/brain injury is different and each person's capacity to heal varies as well. As a result there is "No one size fits all" treatment plan or pathway to healing. This book offers suggestions based on the positive results experienced by my husband and our family during his recovery process. Any therapy or medical treatment discussed in this book was preapproved solely for my husband's use by his medical team.

"But For the Glory of God"
And
All the Survivors of Stroke/Brain Injury
"He" holds in his arms

Acknowledgments

When I walked those long hospital corridors sleep deprived

I would often ask myself, "How on Earth am I still standing?" I walked at a pretty good pace... my shoulders were erect... my back was straight, and I could even produce a smile if I happened to catch eye contact with someone.

Though in retrospect, I know it was the love, support and energy of my family that moved me through our crisis. My inner circle; our children, daughter-in-laws, grandchildren, my mother, sister's, brother, and sister-in-laws; you were there, and met my every need.

Whether you sent me a special song, a bowl of soup or a story to read, I appreciate your intention as you tried to nurture my body, and soul.

You prayed with me and cried with me. You listened through hours of my searching for the right answers. With each conversation I drew from your strength. I was energized by your devotion. I stood strong and steadfast because I had the support of "My Gang." My world is a better place because you're in it.

-I'm so blessed and forever grateful.

About Me, the Author

I was born in Chicago, into a large, middle class family of Polish descent. My earliest thoughts of my future were first and foremost to be a Mom, probably because in my family, someone was always having a baby. The new babies brought joy and excitement, and the women made it look easy.

Other young girls were already aspiring to be teachers, nurses and secretaries; the field of opportunity wasn't huge yet. While none of those other careers interested me, I did say that I thought I would like to manage a business one day. That did raise some eyebrows.

Regardless, all of my dreams came true. We have five wonderful, grown children and have been blessed with six extraordinary grandchildren. My Hospitality career spans thirty years with various management positions in the Hotel and Restaurant Industries.

Today, I'm the Founder/President of "New Normals" a Non-Profit Corporation. My husband's miraculous survival of a severe brain hemorrhage and my role as his caregiver has turned our painful journey into a passion to serve other families, experiencing stroke/brain injury. Our purpose is to provide caregivers, and survivor's informational support and strategies for "Reclaiming a Life of Significance."

We reside in Hanover, Pennsylvania near all of our children and grandchildren.

Contents

Acknowledgments v
About Me, the Author vii

Introduction 1

1   Reservations Required 5
2   Your (Operating Table) is Waiting 11
3   A Test of Faith 15
4   The Guarantee 21
5   One Bad Apple 31
6   Hospital to Rehab 37
7   Let the Healing Begin 47
8   Alpha and Omega 59
9   Designer Therapies 65
10 Prayers and the Specialist 71
11 The Birth of New Normals 77
12 The Paradox-Phenomenon-Plateaus 83
13 All You Need Is Love 89
14 New Year- New Goals 95
15 Saying Good-Bye 101
16 The Goal: "The Speech" 107
17 The Editor 115

About New Normals 121

NEW NORMALS

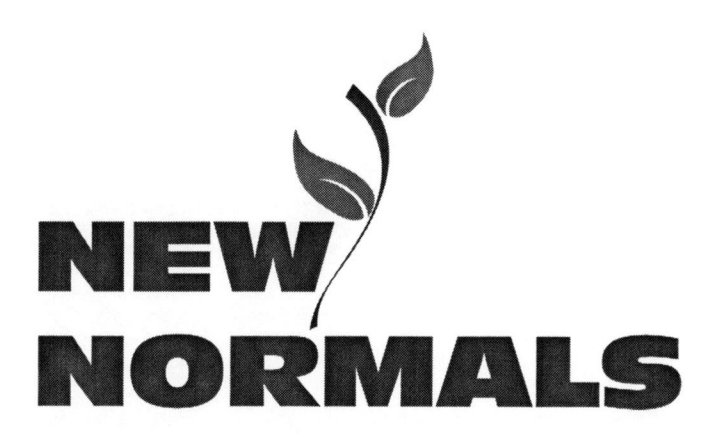

Reclaiming a Life of Significance

Introduction

The number one cause of disability in the United States is due to stroke/brain injury. Every forty five seconds someone suffers a stroke. The statistics are even higher for traumatic brain injury, and are reaching record proportions daily as a by-product of the two wars America faces with Afghanistan and Iraq.

From a layperson's perspective, my knowledge is my first hand experience of stroke/brain injury and it's after effects. Who better to shed light? My experience is recent, and I share an understanding of what happens from that critical moment of the stroke/brain injury that will forever change your life. This book won't eliminate that pain, but I sincerely hope it will help move you through it.

My intention is to serve as an informational guide offering recommendations to improve the healing process; for caregivers, the families, and the survivors of stroke/brain injury.

At the end of each chapter there's a "Best Practices" page of strategies that we employed during my husband's recovery or learned from his process. The majority of these chapters are dedicated to the care of the survivor. I have also addressed our caregiver needs, to nurture our own trauma, and that of our family.

My goal is to encourage your endurance as for some the journey may be long; to be a source of hope if yours starts to diminish, and to offer strategies to stay in faith or regain your faith if you find yourself in times of disconnect.

One of the life altering lessons I learned during this process is the value of words, not only "The Word" of God and its various interpretations, but the words and thoughts we share to comfort each other. Because it's often through the generosity of those that listen…those that understand your plight, that we are rescued. Just the right word at the right moment carries its own healing power.

My first experience with stroke was almost thirty years ago when my maternal grandfather suffered one. "Gramps" was a survivor of Polio. He walked with quite a limp that, I honestly never noticed until a childhood friend asked me, "What's wrong with him?" "Wrong with him," I asked. "Yeah, he walks funny," she said.

Gramps was the happiest man I knew. He had the greatest laugh; loud and full of spirit, just when you thought he was done he'd roll out one more verse. Oh, and it was contagious laughter, soon everyone in the room caught it.

As I entered adulthood, I better understood the challenges he faced all his life with Polio, and grew to admire him even more. He taught us that work was a privilege not to be taken for granted. He more than survived his Polio; he conquered it.

What the Polio may have taken from him was balanced, with an exceptional gift; Gramps knew how to live in the moment. When we went to the lake he'd grab his large black inner tube, and was the first one in the water. At a wedding he was the first one on the dance floor.

By today's standards he would be politely referred to as "disabled." In his lifetime he was referred to as "a cripple." Later in his life, a more sensitive world referred to him as "handicapped." He did eventually succumb to that reference that he was somehow limited, but not until he experienced a stroke. The stroke stole the spirit from him that generated that laughter and dulled his passion for life.

Gramps didn't have the luxury of all the post stroke care thirty years ago that's offered today. No he had Gram, with all her best intentions. A drill sergeant would have been kinder. I think her expectation was that if he could survive the "dreaded Polio" of their day, he could rally from a stroke.

My grandfather's wonderful laughter went silent with the stroke. We never witnessed his crooked walk again, becoming wheelchair dependent he lived only a couple more years. With the standard of care provided today, I believe his survival would have been significantly longer. Simply recognizing the need to treat his depression would have improved his quality of life. The advances in physical therapy might have moved him out of the wheelchair.

My husband and grandfather suffered two different types of strokes. My grandfather's stroke was a non-hemorrhagic, and my husband's stroke produced a severely large hemorrhage. Even with thirty years of improved procedures the survival rate for my husband's hemorrhage are still rare, although great progress has been made, with both types.

After my husband had his stroke, I thought about my grandparents often. I tried to gain insight by remembering their experience, and naturally comparing it to ours. With each memory, I felt grateful for the advances in care. Maybe trying to ease my pain of this difficult time for my grandparents, I chose to remember a happier time. I found myself repeatedly playing in my mind a set of snap shots I had of them dancing together on a hill top. They were each waving top hats, and posed with their beautiful smiles. Somehow even the black and white photo film was able to capture their radiance. They knew how to love and live.

Those pictures were taken probably twenty years before Gramps suffered that stroke. In part I believe my draw to the pictures is the similarity in age; we are about the same age today as they were dancing on that hilltop. It has occurred to me on more than one occasion how fortunate they were to be many years older than we are, experiencing the trauma of stroke/brain injury.

Today the legacy of the pictures holds a greater significance for me; they've become my inspiration to be attentive in my search for joy, and need to have fun. This journey has created a strong desire in me to follow my grandfather's example of living in the moment. In a sense the pictures have spoken, and said, "Woman what are you waiting for?" We have already carefully climbed that mountain "so to speak," these past five years in our healing process- "Reclaiming a Life of Significance."

Yes, indeed it's time. Note to self; next trip, a sunny day, maybe an ocean backdrop, find a hill, climb it and Dance...Dance...Dance. And when "in the moment" I'll turn to my husband, and say, "take your bow Honey, we made it."

CHAPTER 1
Reservations Required

December 25 & 26, 2003

In recent years, The American Stroke Association, has provided an excellent public awareness program on the time sensitive issues associated with stroke; with the signs, symptoms and the slogan: "Time Lost is Brain Lost." The night my husband suffered his brain hemorrhage, I began to question if anyone else had heard this news…

The paramedics arrived to our home within minutes of our "911" call. They proceeded to waste valuable time by suggesting my husband Chris was drunk. "It is Christmas Night," they reminded us. "Or, possibly he has the flu," they suggested. Oh, how I wish it was that simple. When they offered him the option of calling his family doctor in the morning, I wondered who they were looking at. Well, like any macho man my husband began to agree with them. "Enough!" I shouted, "You guys are kidding me right? It was just moments ago he had the classic crushing head pain that moved him out of bed to the floor; he was screaming with pain, his speech is slurred, and his eyes are crossed. "No!" I insisted, "He needs to go to the hospital!"

By the time they reluctantly moved him onto the gurney, and into the ambulance he aspirated on his vomit, and fell into a coma. While they worked frantically to intubate him, their attempts proved unsuccessful. We began transport to the hospital (a five-minute ride) as they bagged him-literally forcing air into his lungs.

Upon arrival, the Emergency Room Physician was waiting for Chris, and was able to quickly intubate him. He was now clinging to life deep in a coma.

The Emergency Room Team moved quickly. With his airway stabilized, blood was drawn and within thirty minutes they completed a CT scan that showed he had a large amount of blood on his brain. The radiologist report suspected a ruptured arterial venous malformation (AVM), possibly a large aneurysm, or a subacranoid hemorrhage.

The hospital staff couldn't have performed more efficiently, until we hit a wall, no Neurosurgeon. We have a critical patient, with a diagnosis. We're in the hospital, they have a Neurosurgeon on staff, but he didn't perform this type of surgery. This particular hospital promoted itself as having a Neuroscience Center; so much for that.

In this state-of-the-art emergency room, surrounded by millions of dollars in equipment, ironically, the most important piece of equipment became the telephone. We needed to get him out of there. He needed surgery, and he had to be transferred to receive it. This local hospital is considered a Level 2 Trauma Center, as are most of our suburban hospitals. He needed to be transferred to a Level 1 Trauma Center.

That night I learned the protocol for the receiving hospital: The Level 1 Trauma Center must have a team in place to accept a patient in need of critical care. I thought, "He needs a reservation, for emergency surgery?" I could not believe what I was hearing. It was Christmas Night, or by that time actually, December 26th. Do you know he was in fact rejected from the first hospital they called? Finally, the second hospital accepted him.

The Emergency Room Nurse assured me this was a better hospital than the first. I'm still confused to this day as to why we wasted so much time waiting on the first hospital. Curiously, neither hospital was the Downtown affiliate to the hospital he was at. Why not place two, three or even four calls at once? Where was the sense of urgency? While every moment mattered, many hours passed...

Under the bright lights of that Emergency Room everything seemed too white, too bright. "What are we doing here? It's Christmas," I thought. How did this happen? For hours on end, I stood in shock at his bedside. I studied his every breath as he lie in his coma. I searched for the energy in his spirit.

Chris is a tall man, with a large frame and muscular build. He possesses a strong presence to match his sum and substance. You knew when my "Honey" entered the room.

In his altered state I wanted desperately to reach him. Gently, I stroked his face, arm and hand. I slipped my trembling hand under his motionless hand, if only for a faint squeeze. I once heard it said that a woman's soul resides inside her heart. No words have ever made more sense to me. In the solitude of those early morning hours, it was my heart that I retreated to. There, I waited to feel him... "Where are you, Chris?"

Many years before, I was with my Dad as he surrendered to death. In those final moments, as he took his last breath, I was able to feel his energy move through me as if to say goodbye... He was leaving. In the presence of Angels, and surrounded by family, we prayed over him as he peacefully transitioned. We then lovingly released him of his pain. "You're safe now Daddy...It's okay, Dad, you can go...We love you Dad."

Now thirteen years later, that familiar sensation found me again, I knew... we were losing Chris. Immediately I was transformed into a wall of resistance. My voice grew loud and strong as I begged, "Please don't leave." In that second I could have moved Heaven and Earth...maybe I did. I felt a surge of energy inside of me. I had the power of a mob of determined women and I used it- waving my hands frantically over him, protecting him and crying, "You're not taking him... Not my husband...You cannot have him... Stay with me Chris... Please don't go... It's too soon.... Please God I can't lose another loved one," I waved my hands and arms over him, until I felt he was safe again.

Two identical feelings, yet so many years apart, each required two totally different responses. Is it possible to defy death, maybe? On some sub-conscious level I believe Chris heard me in that split second, and was reminded to fight. My prayer is that Dad heard us too, in our sacrifice, as we gave him our blessing to leave.

Then my prayers continued. I, too, like so many in that situation made a sacred promise to God. Hospitals have been built in these moments of crisis with God. Some people have committed their lives to the cure of a specific disease or important cause just for the sake of "more time." My prayer was similar; "God just let him live and I promise I will do whatever it takes to bring him back to complete health, and I will teach others what I learn."

This entire process took almost five hours, before the helicopter trauma team had him in the sky transporting him to The University of Chicago Hospital. The Medivac team consisted of a Trauma Doctor, Trauma Nurse and pilot. Chris was in very poor condition at departure. They assured me of his safety, but I couldn't fly with him for insurance reasons. So he would arrive there in eighteen minutes, and I had at least an hour ride by car. I was terrified by our separation.

Best Practices:

1. Beginning the moment of the stroke/brain injury your loved one is unable to make good clear decisions until they heal, care-giving and advocacy begins then.
2. As their advocate, you need to be with them to speak for them if necessary, and supervise their care.
3. Families should set up a schedule, whereby someone is with the patient at all times if possible.
4. Trust your own instincts, if what their telling you doesn't sound right or feel right, they're probably not right.
5. Embrace your faith, and if/so inclined the power of prayer.
6. Start as soon as possible taking notes, you'll be in shock yourself, the notes will proved to be invaluable later.
7. Designate one family member or friend, as the update and information center. This will allow you to focus on your loved one and avoid all the phone calls.

CHAPTER 2
Your (Operating Table) is Waiting

December 26, 2003

Upon arrival at The University of Chicago Hospital, the young Neuro- Surgical Resident greeted me with forms to sign, for what would be Chris' first procedure there. It was the placement of an exterior ventricular drain, to relieve some of the pressure that was building around his brain. He advised me of Chris' grave condition. He went on to express his wish that they had received him earlier and in better shape, but were committed to doing everything within their power.

At first glance of his scans, they weren't sure if Chris had two aneurysms, or a large arterial venous malformation. The remark was, "a very large area of blood from the top of his head to his brain stem." As the drain worked its magic they were better able to see what they were about to operate on, and said it was a large arterial venous malformation of the brain, with a fistula that had ruptured.

We didn't know it at the time, but were fortunate to have one of the World's top-rated Neurosurgeons, perform my husband's surgery, a craniotomy. Chris had an AVM, and this is the doctor, one of few, with the expertise to repair them.

I guess God made Chris' reservation for us that night.

Prior to surgery, his Neurosurgeon did his best to educate me about the procedure, possible outcomes, and chances of survival to follow up care. As he spoke, my focus was split trying to find comfort, a good feeling about this man that I was entrusting my husband's life. I studied his eyes, examined him from head to toe, my thoughts and prayers were racing. "Please bless this man, his hands, his heart, his mind, oh; I hope he had a good night's sleep." I fought to hear him over my pounding heart, and tried to hang on to his every word. Then you graciously entrust your loved one to someone you've known for maybe five minutes. That's all you get.

When he finished preparing me, he asked if I had any questions. "No" I replied, "but... have I told you... how important he is? My husband... His life...is so important to so many...did I tell you how precious he is to me...and Doc... Thank you...I get it... I know the odds aren't in his favor but I trust you, and I know you'll do your best work." He nodded as he said, "We'll get started."

For the months that followed I would remember parts of the conversation from that day, buried deep in my memory, "Yes, he did tell me about this," or "He warned me about that."

By now, the waiting room was filled to capacity with our family. While our youngest daughter moved me from one hospital to the other, our oldest daughter was on the phone waking her brothers. She made their plane reservations and provided them shuttle runs from the airport, to the hospital. We had just celebrated Christmas Eve together hours before. They had all arrived from Maryland and Pennsylvania to Chicago in time for his surgery.

We spent hours quietly waiting together, while he was in surgery. There was nothing left to say. Everyone sat with eyes closed either quietly praying or not wanting to deal with the anguish we all felt. Each time I'd open my eyes, and surveyed the room I'd find one of my beloved children simply staring at me with such sadness, I sent them a wink and a smile as if to say it's going to be alright. Then I withdrew back to that safe place in my heart where my best thoughts originate, and my ongoing conversation with God continued.

After literally hours of waiting, the Neuro Team appeared to review the outcome of the surgery. They felt his surgery was a success, but they were only cautiously optimistic. He had a long road ahead. We were introduced to a possible complication called Vasospasms; these might pose a threat for months to come.

My husband is here, "By the Grace of God," and the dedication of the brilliant Neuro Team at The University of Chicago Hospitals. These doctors commit to advanced studies that most of us are not capable of. This *is* brain surgery. They have mastered skills we take for granted. My prayer is that if you need a Neurosurgeon, your path to them is quick. It was a terrifying road getting Chris into the hands of the right surgeon that night.

Best Practices:

1. With each procedure or surgery request a copy of the Operative Report.
2. You'll need copies of all x-rays and scans as well.
3. Start a folder to collect all handouts and important documents.
4. Start a journal it may bring clarity later.
5. Your daily exercise routine may be interrupted, try to walk for at least 20 minutes each day even if only around hospital grounds. Caregivers, take care of you.
6. Often you can request the medical reports before you leave the hospital and you won't be charged. If you request them after departure there's generally a charge.
7. You don't need the complete hospital record it could be volumes. You'll only need the records that pertain to any doctor or therapist reports for follow up care: Remember-
8. The hospital/ rehabs discharge summary
9. Operative reports
10. Copies of scans or x-rays and the radiology report.
11. Social Service agencies will have their own forms that may need to be filled out by your doctor, but the discharge summary, and the operative reports help provide added information and expedite the process.

Note: The folder that I started that night with the operative reports is still in use today, it is the base of his medical history as it relates to the stroke/brain injury.

CHAPTER 3
A Test of Faith

Sometime between-December 26, 2003 –January 29, 2004

My husband Chris, like so many survivors of stroke/brain injury, enjoyed a healthy and successful life until the moment that artery burst. We, his family, thought he was invincible.

Because, he often traveled for business he was always careful to make the best of his time at home. He would schedule basketball games with our kids, a dinner out with me, a Sunday family dinner, and then back out on Monday. These rituals sustained a decent balance of family life. We enjoyed being together, and made the best of it in support of his career.

Chris is a hard working, highly intelligent man, respected, and admired by many. He is a natural teacher, and his abilities promoted him quickly into Executive Level positions, in the Hospitality Industry. He enjoyed a twenty year run of success, one after the other. We were all so proud of him.

He had a way of teaching our children how to think. I loved to hear him say, "Now... Son... what were you thinking?" Do you know they preferred the wrath of Mom, rather than the calm manner of Dad? I guess thinking is hard when you're a kid.

The hospital became our temporary home for weeks after my husband's brain surgery. The Neuro-Surgical Intensive Care Unit was designed for optimal patient care, not privacy. By design, we all witnessed each other's most private and saddest moments. This was one place where seeing the clergy arrive was not always a comforting experience. The families would gather around the bed with clergy, the window blinds and the door would close. We could hear their muffled cries as they embraced each other, and felt the mood shift of the entire unit. This was a constant reminder of the fragile situation we were in. I tried to take nothing for granted.

In his comatose state the Neuro-Team encouraged communication. For weeks on end I talked, read and sang to him all day, and prayed myself to sleep at night. Each message was filled with love and hope. I reminded him of the times in his life where he was able to walk through, where others sank. I even joked, well sort of; is it a joke if you really mean it? I warned him not to leave me alone with his mother.

His health status fluctuated daily with new infections and complications. It was as though his body was under constant assault.

Born with a sixth sense of sorts, I have learned to trust my instincts. It is the voice in my heart that guides me; I knew Chris would be okay. Usually that was enough for me. But, under this constant stress I couldn't see our future, I was petrified by the present, and the past didn't matter. He was in a coma, breathing by a respirator, had aspiration pneumonia, raging fevers, and was nourished by tubes. He developed a blood clot in his leg. He was on three different antibiotics, and had a drain in his brain…

One afternoon while performing his rounds one of the Resident Neurologists found me at Chris' bedside crying. It was as though the hand of God slapped me on the head. This usually soft-spoken man said to me in an angry voice, "You stop that crying! You stop it right now! He can hear you, what if he sees you? Don't you realize what a GIFT you've been given?" I had no response as he left the room. I was so shaken, if I ever had a reason to cry?

Really, were my tears that offensive to him? Or, truly just an expression of the great sadness I felt watching my husband suffer? Did the doctor misinterpret my tears as a lack of faith? Was it? The Neuro-Team had already nicknamed Chris "The Miracle Man." What did that mean to them? They were always so carefully guarded in their choice of words, often reminding me that he wasn't out of the woods yet. "Complications could arise for months to come," they warned.

Did I have a misperception about Miracles? A Miracle by my definition meant in part, that everything was going to be all right. He had survived an extremely large brain hemorrhage that most don't. Which infection, what tube, kept me from finding comfort in my faith?

When his Neurosurgeon, discussed with me how rare his chances of survival were prior to surgery, I had no doubts. I expected that Miracle. With all the odds against him you still couldn't shake my faith. Each day that he survived, I was humbled by this Miracle. This was the Gift I pleaded for, and received, but I wasn't feeling blessed. I was numb. I had no point of reference. How could I be in the presence of "My God" receiving Miracles and Gifts, and yet be so frightened? This was a true test of faith, unlike anything I had ever known.

When I examined my own thoughts, and the definition of this word "Miracle" it was then, that I was better able to define my beliefs. As with anything in life, I was reminded there's still the element of choice. You can graciously embrace it in its entirety, with absolute faith…or not. The Miracle was his survival; the rest was up to us. The doctor was so right. He is my Gift. This was my turning point. Through him I heard God's voice, felt the slap on the head, and knew "He" was with me... hearing my prayers, "He" was guiding me. The recovery road for Chris was going to be tough and I had to be prepared for it. Temporarily losing my compass, and living without it for even a short period of time was enough to reenergize my faith. How do we measure the depth of our faith, if it's never tested?

No amount of tears, sadness or anxiety was going to change our circumstances. It was time to transform the energy in that hospital room. I needed to protect our Gift, and refocus our future. I needed a plan; I had to start thinking for two. I made a commitment to create a peaceful and healing environment for Chris. He was to be surrounded by love, patience, and positive thoughts. No longer filled with fear, anxiety, and what ifs. I needed to stop approaching each day with fear, because fear was what I was manifesting. I vowed to learn all I could about his illness, and recovery.

I received two gifts that day. Once, I accepted my husband's life as a gift in its unknown and fragile state, I received the gift of knowing that I had the tools and the power within me to bring him through the process. As I moved in faith, my fear slowly subsided. It was replaced with the discovery that all my life experience had prepared me for this moment in time. I either had the answers or the ability to find them. My faith provided me the endurance for his difficult recovery process.

The Bible: Ecclesiastes- Chapter 3:1, 4- To everything there is a season, and a time to every purpose under the heaven: A time to weep, and a time to laugh; a time to mourn, a time to dance...

It would seem to me to be impossible not to weep through this process. The range of emotions that are felt as the brain heals is heart wrenching. There were many tears to dry. The whole family is affected by this illness. As for me, I took the good doctor's advice. When I needed crying time it was private and late at night. Sleep came easy as I was able to recognize, and was comforted by God's fingerprints on our life.

The role as a caregiver to your loved one, a survivor of stroke/brain injury, may be the most important responsibility you'll experience in your lifetime. You can enrich the process by focusing on the marvels that exist within it. Just years ago they hadn't perfected the surgical procedures they use today. The ventilator that I was so terrified of, without this invention my husband wouldn't be here. The feeding tube that sustained him until he could swallow again, or the life saving antibiotics, all gifts of knowledge, all Miracles for inventors, and the millions that benefit from them.

Gaining control of my thoughts and emotions gave me back my hope of finding a happy ending. Embrace with gratitude your place in time, it's not an accident, it is your purpose.

Faith, hope and endurance are the keys to achieving "New Normals."

Best Practices:

1. Begin a gratitude journal, the act of doing this will help you to stay in a positive frame of mind. Can you find five things in each day you're grateful for?
2. Create a family/friend support system to ensure your proper rest. Prepare them for what might happen while you're away and how to react.
3. Learn as much as you can about the illness.
4. Be organized, ask doctors and nurses questions and keep notes.
5. Even a beginner's guide of the brain will help you to understand how it works and possibly point you to the right questions to ask.
6. Progress may seem slow, you need to be patient.
7. Denial is a strong emotion that we sometimes use to protect ourselves until we can cope with the reality of a tough situation. The sooner you're able to embrace the illness/injury the quicker you'll be able to begin to work through it.
8. In the early stages of recovery sleep is vital to the healing process. Don't be alarmed by the amount of sleep. Try to rest when they rest. As they heal the wake time will increase. But, any and all concerns should be discussed, with their doctor or medical team.

CHAPTER 4
The Guarantee

January 2004

My husband's Neurosurgeon has an excellent assistant that handles many details for him. I asked her if she could recommend a book that could help guide me through Chris' recovery process, and her response was an emphatic "NO, There is NO book...you really can't have a book-because every brain heals differently!" I had heard the same line numerous times in the recent weeks, although, I thought she must be mistaken about a guidebook. After all this is The University of Chicago Hospital, they do the research, their doctors develop the procedures. Heck, they should hand you a guidebook as a parting gift.

I went determined into the snow and ice of winter to The University of Chicago Bookstore. Upon the volumes and volumes of brilliantly researched works, I was sure to find my answers. I gave the sales person this long explanation of an arterial venous malformation, fistulas, subarachnoid hemorrhage and craniotomy. I thought for sure there was a step by step guide just waiting for me. Other people surely have survived this...

We diligently searched his computer inventory for my guidebook. Well guess what? There were zero matches for our request. The trip wasn't a complete loss. I did however, leave with a book: *All about the Brain for Dummies*. It described the inner workings of the brain, and its connection to other vital organs. It proved to be a helpful resource that introduced me to this new phase in my life; needing to understand the mysteries of the brain. With my husband in a coma, I had plenty of time to read.

If I had asked for a book about strokes or even possibly a book on traumatic brain injury, I may have had some luck. But, as they were so specific to his diagnosis, I thought in order to get the right book I needed to be precise as to his condition. I didn't know that an arterial venous malformation of the brain is considered a hemorrhagic stroke. And remember I was already told that there is "NO" book.

Stroke/Brain injury is the number one cause of disability in the United States. After much research on the different types and causes it can be simplified by two categories. They are Acquired Brain Injury (ABI) and Traumatic Brain Injury (TBI).

Examples of Acquired Brain Injury (ABI) include stroke, brain tumors, brain cancers, aneurysm, arterial venous malformations, and brain infections, near suffocation, drug overdose or carbon monoxide poisoning. Under the umbrella of stroke there are several different types of stroke as well; the two most common references are the hemorrhagic strokes (the bleeders) and the non-hemorrhagic (the ischemic).

Examples of Traumatic Brain Injury (TBI) are the result of motorcycle, car, bike accidents, gunshot wounds, falls, sports injury, assaults and an unfortunate by product of war. Traumatic Brain Injury is usually prefaced with a rating scale from mild to severe.

Common physical changes experienced by some survivors following stroke/brain injury- These injuries may be short term or long term:

1. Motor Skills
2. Balance Impairments
3. Hearing Loss
4. Vision Loss
5. Speech Disorders
6. Communication
7. Swallow Disorders
8. Tremors
9. Spasticity
10. Ataxia
11. Fatigue
12. Weakness
13. Seizures
14. Paralysis
15. Loss of Taste and Smell

Common changes in cognition and thinking experienced by some survivors following stroke/brain injury-These injuries may be short term or long term:

1. Loss of long and/or
2. Short term memory
3. Attention Deficits
4. Speed of Information Processing
5. Receptive and Expressive Aphasia
6. Problem Solving
7. Organizational Skills

8. Self Perception
9. Cognitive Impairments
10. Decreased Awareness
11. Depression
12. Social and Emotional Problems

The recovery process can take weeks, months or years depending upon the degree of injury. The normal course of treatment begins in the hospital emergency room then moves to a stroke or intensive care unit. Some hospitals today provide a Neuro- Intensive Care Unit. Generally there's a step down phase of hospitalization to the Neuro or Stroke Floor as the patient continues to stabilize. The patient is then moved to a rehab center. Some brain injuries may require extended nursing facility care, and many will go home. Often in home care/therapy services will begin until the patient is ready for outpatient rehab services.

The expertise of numerous medical professionals may be necessary throughout the recovery process.

The Rehab Specialist:

1. Neurosurgeon
2. Neurologist
3. Neuro-Psychologist
4. Physical therapist
5. Occupational therapist
6. Speech/swallow therapist
7. Primary Care or Internal Medicine Physician
8. Psychiatrist
9. Vocational Counselor
10. Case Managers/Social Workers

11. Physiatrists/Rehabilitation MD
12. Respiratory Therapist
13. Neuro- Ophthalmologist
14. Ear Nose and Throat MD
15. Recreational Therapist
16. Nutritionist

The list of possible outcomes/disabilities and therapeutic needs in itself demonstrates why one of the first conversations with medical personnel post injury will unfold with similarity- "Each stroke/brain injury is different. Each brain heals differently." While there may be a reasonable amount of certainty as to when the swelling in the brain will subside, the extent of the damage to, or pathways to healing, will remain unclear, and not promised. To endure this healing process with its inherent uncertainty often leads to isolation and hopelessness.

When I'm lost I'll stop and ask for directions, I don't like to waste time. When I managed hotels we had a business plan. Even raising our five children, while at times we wish they came with instructions, we had our life experience that we drew wisdom from, and plenty of opinions for the asking.

In my world I like to believe that there's a solution for every problem. I soon came to realize that I was complicating things. Because I not only wanted solutions, I wanted guarantees. That if we performed this procedure or followed a certain course of therapy that we could expect a positive result, and there were no promises. Not every story had a happy ending.

Trying to keep in mind no one is promised tomorrow, we did our best to control today. Chris has endured years of therapy to date and he's the first one to say, "It is what it is... until it changes."

On Thanksgiving Day, we have a family tradition where we go around the table and each person shares what they're most grateful for. I'm usually very long winded, but this particular year I said only that, "I was grateful for the prayers that were answered, and grateful too for the prayers that were not answered." There was a long pause of silence at the table. Some may have politely thought I lost my place. While others thought "She can't possibly be done, not our Mom." The silence was broken when I heard... "Huh? Mom, what do you mean?" I replied, "I'm not confused-We've all heard the line-be careful what you wish for?" Haven't you ever wished or prayed for something, and later said, "Thank God," that didn't happen. I choose to believe there's a reason when my prayers aren't answered. I accept it and know that it wasn't in my best interest.

Today, I'm glad I didn't know what type of book to ask for at The University of Chicago Bookstore. They may have sold me a book on strokes/brain injury that might have sufficed my need at that time. Instead my journey, and search for answers exposed me to a different realm of thoughts. They all said, "too different-heals different"- lead me on a search of questioning, "Where's the similarities, what's the same?"

To my surprise, and among all the differences emerged all the commonalties. It's in the after affects, the "recipe for renewal": all of our families have suffered the pain of watching their loved one struggle to survive. I believe we have common bonds, as survivors of stroke/brain injury, their caregivers, and the people that love them. It's in the feelings we share, and while there are few guarantees with this process, I can guarantee this- someone is dealing with some of the same things you are- someone else is fighting through the same feelings you have- they may feel vulnerable-they may feel sad sometimes. Why is it so important to know this? Because, it eliminates the mystery and isolation of the challenge, if we know someone else feels this too.

Many experience financial difficulties. We have fear of meeting our future needs. There's the stress on relationships, families, and marriage. By sharing our experience with each other we empower and support.

Through our stories we co-create hope for the future. Just knowing "If he can make it, I should too - If she survived that I can too." They said he would never walk again, he'd always have a tracheotomy and be fed by a tube-he refused to quit, and look at him now.... We can share our hope, faith and vision.

Outside the perimeter of feelings there are common functional disabilities experienced by both categories, whether the origin of injury is from an ABI or TBI, and depending on severity, as seen in the lists on previous pages. The same therapists and physicians for both, guide the renewal processes. Don't allow all the different terminology to become confusing. All you need is a diagnosis and a treatment plan.

At the end of the day the best guidebook for me was *The Bible*. As I prayed for guidance, I stood tough to the test.

Best Practices:

1. Join a stroke support group and/or a caregiver support
2. Some states offer special programs from their office on aging that will provide family support and aide.
3. Seek marriage counseling if necessary to cope with all the changes.
4. This is a family affair. Is counseling in order? Do your kids need the support of a school guidance counselor/ or a school psychologist?
5. Reach out to your church/synagogue or clergy for guidance.
6. Have family meetings to allow all to express their feelings.
7. Involve all family members in the recovery process, it helps to be a part of a solution
8. Remind them that you've created an atmosphere of healing and they need to leave their problems and sadness at the door.
9. Protect your home-it needs to be a place of positive and peaceful thoughts.

"Recipe for Renewal"

Serves many well -No need to bake- Repeat daily
May store at room temperature

<u>Gently Fold</u>:
    2- pounds- Hope
    2- pounds- Faith
    2-pounds- Endurance

<u>Sift:</u>
    2-heaping teaspoons- Laughter
    5- pounds- Patience
    4- pounds- Prayer

<u>Blend</u>:
    2- quarts-Exercise
    5- pints-Fresh Air
    3- portions-Good Nutrition

<u>Shake Don't Stir</u>:
    1- pound- Music
    2- cups-Sunshine
    3- handfuls-Joy

<u>Mix Well</u>:
    1- cup-Unconditional Love
    1- cup-Positive Thoughts
    1- cup-Gratitude

<u>Toss:</u>
    2- tablespoons-Goals
    2- tablespoon- Dreams
    2- tablespoon- Passion

<u>Optional Topping:</u>
    2- dashes-Determination
    1- pinch- Blessings
    4-sprinkles-Expectations

CHAPTER 5
One Bad Apple

September 2003-September 2008

For months I had an internal debate about sharing our hospital/rehab experiences in this guide. As my memory unfolded in each page it became abundantly clear, that it would be impossible for me to separate. The multitude of times that I was forced to be my husband's voice, and protect him often arose inside the hospital walls. My commitment to a better tomorrow for survivors of stroke/brain injury must begin in these hospitals. This information must be communicated to promote correction.

I have tried to teach my kids the value of learning from a negative experience, as these were some of my best lessons. It's my intention to teach others what we learned, and hopefully protect someone from a dangerous situation.

I have withheld the names of all the hospitals/rehab involved, with the exception of The University of Chicago Hospital as they provided the best experience. I'm far too grateful for my husband's life, and each provided a role in saving it. Also, it is my belief these same problems exist in, "Any Hospital USA".

Do you know with every problem I encountered I was never prepared for the possibility of the next one- I felt like a car being side swiped at each turn. We were fighting for his life and more times than I like to remember, I was battling to get him appropriate care.

Over the years my personal hospital experience has been limited to short stays for childbirth, and minor procedures. I can honestly say I had relatively pleasant experiences. Staffs were caring and friendly. You received your medicine, meals and procedure, with skill then it's time to go home.

Our five-year journey began a few months prior to Chris' brain surgery. We had a brief encounter, with the healthcare system when my mother in law fell, and broke her hip and leg. It was a nightmare communicating, and traveling between Florida and Illinois until she was strong enough for us to move her. The hospital followed by the nursing/rehab facility she was in, was horribly understaffed.

Her longtime physician disagreed with our decision to move her, and worse, encouraged her continued independence from us. At that time she was 88 years old, had serious osteoporosis, osteoarthritis, difficulty hearing even with hearing aids, and was recently diagnosed legally blind due to macular degeneration. She was in a meeting at the Lighthouse for the Blind, learning to cope with her blindness, when she tripped over a chair leg and fell.

Under the circumstances, we were very grateful that someone was there with her when it happened. Yet, her doctor felt after a month in a nursing home, and therapy she could live alone. With a home health care agency to check on her a few days a week, he thought she would be fine. What if she didn't hear the doorbell, or couldn't see whom she was inviting into her home? She was now in a wheelchair, no family nearby, and could barely hold her head up from the pain medicines; I thought you've got to be kidding me. I couldn't believe my ears. Was this all about a paycheck?

When it's said the healthcare system is broken, it's not just a surly nurse, or long waits, or a dirty bathroom that people are complaining about. Chris has been in numerous hospitals since the stroke and rehab. As we managed my mother-in-law's illness and Chris' illness simultaneously, this chapter, and my recollections throughout this book are based on my experience. It spans a five-year period with numerous hospitals, nursing facilities, rehab centers- in and out patient care, same day surgical centers, private doctors, and therapists, as well.

Our story begins that Christmas Night. With what I believe was an obvious lack of education about stroke symptoms from the First Responders: The Emergency Technicians. They wasted no time getting to us. They arrived ready, willing and able to save a life. However, that's where the good news ends-they were obviously unaware of what to look for.

Our local Level 2 hospital should have had a system in place to expedite the patients that they knew they can't provide service for. I don't believe the ER Doctor enjoyed waiting for a phone call that night, nor the nurse as we watched Chris slip away.

You would think the hospitals would be lined up waiting for him. He was insured, and his medical bills totaled hundreds of thousands of dollars in the first few months alone.

I don't think my mother-in-law's doctor wanted to harm her intentionally, but it only took commonsense to see she was unable to care for herself, not a medical degree. Maybe he was too busy to understand the complete scope of what he was suggesting.

My husband was in two highly respected hospitals that night. Both have won numerous awards, and they continue to enjoy numerous awards each year with top rankings. The rehabilitation hospital he was in, held a top ranking as well. By some standards we were the lucky ones, living near a big city, and to have so many choices in a sixty mile radius. But if they don't have an action plan for the patients they are incapable of providing service for, the system fails. They must communicate.

Then there were the Nightingales, probably 98% of the nurses are terrific, caring, knowledgeable professionals that are committed to their patients. They saved me many nights as Chris would wake and try to jump out of bed. Why aren't we talking them up more? Why does the other 2% get so much press? I suppose the shear nature of the profession. The life and death situation they face daily forces them under the microscope. We require so much more from them than the average profession.

We were very fortunate to have a terrific Intensive Care Unit Nurse the first few days after Chris' craniotomy. He was her only patient, and she fussed over him all day. She set the standard of care for him in my mind. I expected he would receive this same care each day.

Unfortunately, not every nurse addressed his needs as she did. I'm the first one to give someone the benefit of doubt, making excuses for him or her that they're in an over worked system. However, I have been witness to an ICU nurse, with a one to one ratio for care that barely moved all day. Even some of the best hospital systems have that 2% ratio.

There is an undeniable human factor here. Some people simply have poor work ethics. Most will do the right thing with little or no supervision, while others only move when their supervisor is in sight, purely a matter of integrity. I've found incompetence at every level, and a system that's at the mercy of sometimes incompetent or burned out nurses, because of the nursing shortage.

The following suggestions come from my own personal contact with the medical community in four states with two different patients over a five-year time frame.

Best Practices:

1. If you encounter an incompetent nurse or other medical personnel be specific and report the problem.
2. Address your problems with the hospital or nursing facility head on. I found that hospital administrators are generally attentive and concerned.
3. Most facilities have a manager on duty type program twenty four hours a day-use it
4. Whether caseworkers, social workers, a patient advocacy program, each hospital offers some form of communication to resolve problems, it just has different titles.
5. They would prefer if you resolve your issues with them before calling a JACHO, (the governing and licensing board for hospitals.)
6. I found nurse managers are a good source and resource of information.
7. Insist that they provide the proper standard of care.
8. Embarrass them into doing the right thing if you have to. Remind them of the hospital's marketing promise; they all have one "Excellence in Care," "The promise to exceed all expectation." Let them know that's the standard you expect.
9. The key when you're in the trenches so to speak is to find ways to make the system work for you. Ask questions, know the patient's rights.
10. My best advice, stay alert. If you're loved one is in serious condition and unable to make their own decisions – do not leave them alone.

11. They need an advocate. Sort it out with family-take a leave of absence, whatever it takes to have a family member with that patient.
12. You can request to stay twenty four hours a day. Most hospitals will give you a rollaway bed or at least a decent chair to sleep in.
13. Call your insurance company and lodge your complaints, make them aware of the sub-standard care you're receiving.
14. Later tell your story and put pressure on your insurance plan administrator. They pay the policy; they negotiate the terms each year.
15. If you're truly concerned about a specific nurse or attendant's care, request that they no longer be assigned to your loved one.
16. Some hospitals have a hotline for complaints
17. Use your voice-become a letter writer. Each hospital has a board of directors.
18. Some have a hotline directly to the hospital's corporate office to prevent your potential JACHO calls
19. Have your family lawyer make a call-they'd rather hear from them now, rather than later. This allows the facility time to correct the issues. That's all you really want, better care.

CHAPTER 6
Hospital to Rehab

January 29, 2004 -March 6, 2004

My husband wasn't allowed to wake completely from his coma until his first evening in the rehab hospital. His Neuro Team kept him in a medically induced semi comatose state, to allow him more time to heal. They did try to wake him a few times, and found a raging bull. Back down he went, but in that semi state it was a little less lonely. He could squeeze my hand on command. He could nod or wink when I told him I loved him. He could open his eyes for a few minutes at a time. We saw real progress when they took the catheter out of his bladder, and he could motion for the urinal bottle. We'd just hand it to him and he could manage it under the covers somehow, and hand it back to us full. Never spilling a drop, and never opening his eyes. My sister is a nurse, and we thought for sure that this was a positive sign.

I chose the rehabilitation hospital by reputation, even though it was highly ranked, in the "top ten" statewide. I did interview the number one ranked rehab hospital. When I inquired into their nursing care, the caseworker was rather dismissive, and stated we all have the same nursing problems. She was too quick to accept their inadequacy. I asked Chris' Neurosurgeon which one he recommended and he stood by the outstanding program at number one. However, he said that other would be adequate, and the added benefits to the family of being closer to home would outweigh any differences. It was winter in Chicago.

As he woke from his coma, Bernadette his new evening nurse guided me as to my tone. "Speak to him softly and slowly for now," she said. She read his chart and history sent over from the hospital, and proceeded to ask me questions about her patient, not the usual medical stuff. She wanted to know all about him. Who was he before this happened, what did Chris do, career, hobbies, his roots, and our family? It was so nice to have a real conversation and remember him.

Bernadette was nearing retirement age, with lovely, long, silver hair, always worn up. She was a straight shooter, smart and wise. She spoke with a strong German accent, and maneuvered her reassuring smile from patient to patient. This woman loved her work.

They didn't waste any time when he arrived at the rehabilitation hospital. His therapies began the next morning. Barely out of his coma, they moved him, and accessed him. Not uncommon from a brain injury, he woke very agitated. He could hardly speak, and with great difficulty, maybe you could make out a word here or there. He had a tracheotomy, but what we didn't know at that point, was there was damage to his vocal cords as well.

When they suggested he try to write we realized he had vision problems. He wrote each word on top of the other. With some coaching we taught him to move the pen after each word. Most times he made sense, this was a good sign. He was six weeks post brain surgery when he arrived for rehab. He had what was considered profound dysphasia-he couldn't swallow. He still had some pneumonia from the aspiration. His body was so weak from the weeks in a coma; he had lost forty pounds, and had no muscle tone. With that his strength was lost, as was his ability to stand or walk, and he fell to the side, if you tried to sit him up. It still takes my breath away as I write this, thinking about his condition.

For his protection they assigned him an aide twenty fours hour a day. These aides provided one on one simple care. Their biggest challenge was to prevent him in his agitated state from pulling out his G-tube, the tube that fed him directly into his stomach, or worse his trachea tube.

We got off to a very rocky start at rehab.

Day 1- They insisted I went home to sleep each night. I was so tired and ready for my own bed, but he had awakened from the coma lost and confused. No one could understand him, and he was calmed only by my presence. We agreed I would stay until he went to sleep. I could call the nurse's station any time to check on him, and could arrive back as early in the morning as I desired, until he adjusted to his new environment.

Day 2- I was in the Nurse Manager office as they had tied his hands in restraints during the night. No one called me as promised if he had problems in the night. There is a form you can sign that disallows the practice of restraints; it was conveniently given to me after the event.

Day 3-The Ear Nose and Throat Doctor during his swallow evaluation said it could be as long as a year that Chris would need the trachea tube. He had never witnessed such profound dysphasia, and he also suffered from bilateral vocal cord paralysis. "He may always need the trachea tube and the G-tube to feed him. He probably sustained brain damage to his Vagus nerve." Rather than allowing him to continue his prophesy of gloom and doom, and as Chris grew more agitated, I tried to take control of the conversation. "Well," I interrupted, "We will need to consult with other specialist in this area. Honestly Doc, this entire conversation may be premature as my husband is barely out of his coma, it's only been three days." The good doctor obviously did not like having his expertise questioned. In a very sarcastic and loud tone he replied, "You know his inability to swallow is the least of his problems." Chris wasn't deaf he heard him and understood him. I guess he was more aware than the doctor realized. I met the Director of the Swallow Clinic that day, and lodged a complaint.

Day 4-As I mention the last two weeks in the hospital Chris was able to urinate, with frequency and accuracy into the plastic urinal bottle, in a semi comatose state. I know it was real, I emptied the bottle, and he'd almost fill it. My sister was a witness; it was one of our first rays of hope in his recovery. Well suddenly I'm told he has a problem with lack of urination. They started to discuss the need for intermittent catheterization to empty his bladder and if it didn't improve, he would need surgery. The doctor insisted this procedure was often necessary after brain injury and they were capable of performing at their facility. I believe the doctor was telling me the truth it just didn't make any sense to what I had seen in recent weeks, something was wrong.

Later Day 4-I found myself in the Chapel on my knees. This can't be happening. My Mom's words came to me as I prayed, she often says, "I'm between a sweat and a tear." She has raised my sister's three kids since she passed several years ago, and never complains of the difficult situation she is in. Instead she reminds me that they are her reason to wake up every day. But, from time to time I try to force a deeper conversation I'll ask "how are you really doing Mom?" Her response is always the same, "Oh, between a sweat and a tear. Yes... a sweat and a tear." She sighs. I get it Mom...

Day 5-That morning I started to question the day nurse and doctor as to the amount of water he was getting by G-tube. The only and probably the greatest difference is he had an IV of fluids at the hospital, plus his liquid feedings, and water by G-tube. I explained the whole scenario of his ability to urinate at The University of Chicago Hospital. They looked at me with disbelief. "He's getting two hundred cc's of water at each feeding," his nurse said. She made it sound like that was a lot.

It just kept getting worse. Later that day Chris was trying to tell me his night aide Marta was threatening to cut him. He was so frustrated I couldn't understand him, and I didn't want to believe what he was saying. Cut you? –I was losing friends pretty quickly there. I was ready to place him in the car and drive him home. When his evening nurse Bernadette came in we tried to make sense of the whole thing, we questioned Marta. "Can you think of any words you might say to him that sound like cut?" She looked so frightened; she did have a strong Spanish accent. And he appeared genuinely frightened of her too. This was real. I tried to decide what to do; Bernadette said Marta was one of their best employees. As she went back to work she asked Bernadette if Chris had urinated yet, and proceeded to say, "I'll have to **cath** him," with that accent it sounded an awful lot like **cut**. One problem solved.

At his next feeding, I asked Bernadette to show me how to feed him. When I saw how little two hundred cc's of water was I knew the problem...it's only seven ounces of water! I filled baby bottles with eight ounces. I learned the metric system quickly that day. He was scheduled for surgery in the morning.

Day 6-Began with a screaming match between me, the doctor, and the morning nurse. The resolution was, he was to have his fluids increased immediately, and we would give it forty eight hours to determine any further procedures. The doctor wanted twenty four hours, I said, "absolutely not he's probably partially dehydrated from the lack of fluids the past few days." I took responsibility for making sure he got his water that day, and at day's end he was urinating normally.

Before, I left that night I gave instruction that this procedure of intermittent catheterization was never to be performed again without my approval.

Day 7-It was time to learn whatever I could and prepare to take him home. The nursing staff was great even the one I disagreed with. The therapists were terrific and worked so hard with him. But, I had serious problems with the two physicians assigned to him. I learned to take advantage of the best of what they offered and found ways to manage the rest. Truly, in these settings the doctors have the least amount of contact with the patients- that made it easier to manage.

The best part of the day was the evening and Bernadette. Chris felt safe with her and looked forward to her daily arrival. Sometimes she would come in before her shift and check up on him while he was in therapy. She cheered with us when he took his first step holding on to the parallel bars.

He took a nap each day after therapy, and when she realized the amount of time I spent there she encouraged me to share his bed, and take a nap with him. "Just draw the curtain" she'd say, finally permission to do something normal.

From a complicated illness, and its inherent caution signs Bernadette ease of the situation gave me valuable insight. You're no longer fearful of a tube when you understand its purpose, and better yet, how to reinsert it if it falls out. The creation of providing a more normal environment only occurred when I gained the knowledge of caring for his basic physical needs.

Every evening she told me stories of the brain injuries she witnessed over years, the success stories. In her way she did her best to prepare me for length of time his recovery would take. While I mentally rejected her reference to the possibility of "years of recovery"-I listened politely. And when Chris' recovery took longer than I anticipated I went to my memory searched for her words, and used them to console myself. "There was still time to hope," I'd say to myself.

When my eyes weren't solely on Chris and I observed the other patients in the rehab, it became painfully obvious that Chris was in terrible shape compared to most.

I also realized we exhausted the expertise of the doctors there. He was a pretty complicated case. He needed more specialized care for his vocal cords, dysphasia, and eye care. My gut told me just waiting for the vagus nerve to heal, as suggested, was not his answer. The rehabs original action plan for him changed, with the ENT's diagnosis of profound dysphasia, and bilateral vocal cord paralysis. His first care plan goal included the removal of the trachea tube in a few weeks. The new plan was to perform speech and swallows exercises with a "wait and see" approach. That wasn't acceptable.

I made a list of his injuries that resulted from the hemorrhage. Writing it down helped me to recognize where some opportunities to speed up the process might be. Knowing him, and how important the simple act of eating would be for his overall health, well-being and enjoyment; we focused our search for a vocal cord specialist. If we could cure this one injury, I hoped for a domino effect, then swallow would improve, trach could be removed, and the feeding tube.

After one month I told his caseworker it was time for me to take him home. Chris' case worker tried to talk me out of removing him early; they already had him approved through the insurance for another month of rehab care or more if needed.

Then she bluntly told me she didn't think I could handle him, and it would be a mistake for me to try. "He has too many disabilities. Normally in these situations we could show you by providing a trial home visit, but even that's not possible because he needs too much supportive equipment."

What she failed to realize, according to their current care plan for him he would need that same equipment for months or maybe forever. So thirty or sixty more days would provide what, more of the same? That was not an option.

Well, better have bullied me, without a flinch I explained my reasoning. "I have been preparing for a month to take him home, and I have learned how to:

1. Suction his trach- they wanted him to learn to do this but his eyesight was too poor.
2. Change the trach
3. Feed him through the G-tube
4. Clean the tube and its surrounding area
5. Bathe him and wash his hair while protecting his airway.
6. Operate all the respiratory equipment and his oxygen
7. I didn't miss a therapy session during his stay here and kept a file.
8. Administer his medicines
9. He would start Home Care immediately-Speech-Physical-Occupational therapies.

10. Insurance allows a few nursing visits each week and my sister is a nurse.

11. I'll have part-time support of our two daughters-both young adults
12. I found an Internist that just moved her practice to the suburbs and committed to taking him as her patient. She agreed to be available by phone whenever I needed her.

"The main reasons I'm moving him early are; first, this is what Chris wants. Second, I now know I can provide the same standard of care but in a more positive, comfortable atmosphere. Finally, it's time to get him the specialized care he needs to advance to a new level. And they won't allow my pursuit of outside specialists to come to this facility, nor transporting him to theirs, so really if he stays here we're holding him back."

It took another week to get all the necessary equipment sent to the house, set up a home care agency, and schedule. The rehab graciously provided me with a complete folder of information from emotional issues that may arise, to where to purchase his liquid meals. They were very professional about his departure, and worked hard to ease his transition. Upon departure they reminded me that I could bring him back if I found caring for him at home was too difficult.

We needed to install assistive devices in our bathrooms. Prepare a chart for all his medications. It was March and the Christmas tree was still up! I had the house deep cleaned including the carpet. There was a lot to do, soon it would be Easter and springtime was just around the corner.

Best Practices:

1. Weigh your options, and ask yourself, is the current care situation the best care plan. I would never encourage- anyone to leave good care early, unless their needs were not being met. (My husband is a complicated case that required specialized care that he was not receiving.)
2. To begin to create a normal environment you need to be able to offer or reintroduce the familiar, and that won't happen in a hospital or rehab setting.
3. Learn to interview doctors and therapists explain the scope of patients needs to them, and ask if they feel they can provide those services for you. Write all your questions down prior to interview.
4. For them to make a good assessment they will need a clear past history. Offer to provide them with the medical records for their review.
5. Don't be afraid to say, NO! Don't let anyone bully you if you know you're right.
6. Don't allow anyone to limit you ("you can't handle him") when you know you can accomplish something.
7. No matter how difficult the situation or problems try to engage them in helping you.
8. Develop the plan for after care, before you bring your loved one home.
9. Stay humble, it's about the patient not about ego's or personalities.

CHAPTER 7
Let the Healing Begin

March 6, 2004- To present day

He finally came home after ten weeks in hospitals. He was exhausted, and needed a nap as soon as we arrived home. He was happy to be back in our king-size bed. When he woke he said that was the best nap he ever had. Ahhh...Praise for the familiar.

I reminded him of when he woke from his coma terrified and confused; I made him a promise that together we would find his way back. "That begins today"...

My husband told me once, years prior to his injury, "I don't know where I begin and end or where you begin and end; our lives are so intertwined." His words spoke so true to me when he couldn't speak at all. Somehow I was the only one that understood him. It was his voice in my head, his worrier voice. I can remember feeling almost panicked by some of the consequences of the brain hemorrhage. I wanted to protect him. I feared how he would handle his drooling, or his misguided paralyzed tongue. This was a devastating dichotomy from the man my husband was pre-brain injury, to the man post injury. I knew he would be horrified by his condition.

The blessing lies in what he couldn't comprehend yet. I was grateful that he was generally unaware of some of the after effects caused by the brain injury, until he was strong enough to deal with it. As for me, I able to kiss him through his drool, and was thankful for his presence.

For him, and I pray for other's going through a similar experience, it was as though there was special protection in place. He didn't realize his drooling or the lack of control with his tongue nor, could he really see it. By the time he regained more vision and mental clarity, the therapies had improved both issues.

Seeing God's fingerprints along the journey made it bearable. So often things that I thought would be difficult for Chris to face, he never had to. It was two years before he realized how crossed his eyes were. It took everything I had not to laugh when one morning he said to me, "I never realized how screwed up my eyes are."

Even though he was fed only by a tube directly into his stomach for months, he never felt hungry or thirsty, how could this be if not for "God's Grace?"

Although, I was saddened by how blunted his feelings were, today my testimony would be complete gratitude. He was never truly happy, and never severely depressed. Rather than addressing a wide range of feeling or emotions, his time was best spent recovering from each individual injury.

Hospitals provide all the critical care necessary to keep you alive. Rehabs provide the strategies needed to recover. Home is where healing begins. Before I brought him home I made a list of his current disabilities, and had an action plan for each. In the process of drafting the list, by comparison, it was close only to birth, and the first year of development. His rebirth process included lists of dos and don'ts for dealing with the survivor of a brain injury; important ways to prevent undesirable behaviors or meltdowns from over stimulation.

Prior to leaving the rehab center we had a few sessions with their Neuro-Psychologist to identify, and address his emotional problems that resulted from the brain injury. I also met with her alone to learn, and devise a plan for our family to employ with consistency. He woke agitated with impulsivity issues-which are defined as a lack of self-control, and poor judgment. Significant to his recovery process would be an understanding of his emotions, and how to best manage them.

While I cover many items in this chapter as a general rule for creating a healing environment, it may not encompass all the needs for your loved one. Again, there's not a one size fits all stroke/brain injury recovery method. But it is a good base, and you can incorporate the needs significant to their healing process.

After ten weeks of uncertainty between the coma, and unknowns of hospital- rehabs, he was home and healing. Our five grown, very devoted children needed to be released from their daily worries. Determined to create a more normal environment for all of us, it was time to gently nudge them out of his sick bed, and back to life...

Our kids are thick as thieves, and armed with an efficient grapevine system. I needed a clear repetitive message. My five discussions went something like this: "Your Dad is my responsibility; he would never want to be a source of worry or sadness in your life. It's time to start a new chapter. You could never hurt enough or cry enough to change his outcome. Please pray and stay focused on things or ideas that might bring him pleasure. Be positive and send positive energy his way. That's what we need most from you now." Feeling isolated from them at times, it was difficult to not draw them back in.

Best Practices:

1. **Essential Environment-**
   - A daily structure/schedule is imperative. It will be of comfort to them to know what comes next, what they can expect. Try to avoid disruptions in the daily plan it will cause confusion and unnecessary stress.
   - Create a Chaos Free Zone- free of loud or excess noise, free of multiples, example: radio on, stereo on, TV on, everyone talking at once. Controlling the environment will help avoid the over-stimulation and feelings of being overwhelmed. Creating a positive secure environment will promote healing.
   - Make your home an extension of the therapy office/rehab. Your therapist will assign you homework. Schedule your home programs as you do your appointments for better continuity.
   - We had a Home Team, our oldest daughter helped with speech homework and the trach, our youngest daughter paid bills and ran errands, our granddaughter only age 5 at the time, played balloon volleyball with my husband when he was wheelchair dependent.
   - Even his sister that lived in a different state was able to help, each morning she would surf the internet sports pages, find stories of interest, increase the font large enough for Chris to see it easily, then email it to him for his daily eye exercises. She was also a huge help with research.

- My sister is a Registered Nurse and she guided his care nightly by phone, and visited a couple of times a week.
- I filled in all the gaps, and focused hours, weeks, months, and years on rebuilding his speech. I also had the task of carefully addressing some of his behaviors-it was very difficult to correct him in a positive manner.
- Everyone was able to participate in recreational therapies, all family even the grandchildren. Mostly we played board games. This was very important because it helped to rebuild his attention span or was used as a diversion on tougher days.
- All living space should be organized and clean. Create an orderly system by placing, example: mobility aids, medication, and therapy material-equipment in the same place every time; this will help to eliminate accidents and prevent the frustration of trying to find it when you need it.
- Rest periods throughout the day are of vital importance.

2. **Encouragement-**
    - Surround yourself with people that will be supportive positive and uplifting. If you know your brother Harry has a tendency to say all the wrong things but has good intentions- limit or avoid visits. However refocus his good intentions to benefit you in some way- maybe he could take the car to be serviced or run errands- mow the lawn. Let him be a blessing to you.

- Many people sent cards, some wonderful letters describing how my husband's life motivated and inspired them. We kept a folder and I read them to him often as a reminder of how important he is.
- It was a difficult time for our 3 sons because we just moved from Maryland to Chicago. The separation was difficult for all of us-and further complicated by his illness- the vocal cord paralysis and the trach prevented communication. I needed to find a way for our son's, friends and other family members to express encouragement. While still in rehab I requested permission to put an answering machine on Chris' room phone. The only potential problem the rehab center had was if a phone constantly ringing could be upsetting to other patients. So I turned the ringer off and left a message to all callers that we appreciate their call, suggested they leave a message. Each evening Chris and I would listen to his messages it was a great way to end each day. We continued this same practice when we arrived home as well.
- At home we created a rehab/exercise area for Chris. On the walls in this room we hung all of Chris' favorite family pictures, his favorite motivational sayings and displayed awards he had earned over the years. Positive reminders are everywhere- in our bathroom- just above the sink we have a wall plaque that says-"Never- Never Give Up". It's our first reminder each day.

- We constantly encouraged his progress no matter how small. Soon, progress was more significant.

3. **Education-**
    - Learn all you can about your health issue take notes and bring questions to gather as much information from each visit.
    - Use your local libraries and Internet
    - When using the Internet use searches for stroke and brain injury.
    - The American Stroke Association has a useful website and free magazine. www.strokeassociation.org
    - The National Stroke Association as well has a useful website and a free magazine-we belong to both. www.stroke.org
    - AAPD- American Association of People with Disabilities-offers a quarterly newsletter on latest in legislation to improve the lives of people with disabilities. There's a small membership fee. www.aapd.com
    - The most complete guide I've read to date is: *Dr. Joel Stein's-Stroke and the Family- a New Gui*de. The appendix has numerous resources, information and websites.
    - Rehab centers can usually provide you with handouts on some specific ailments.
    - Ask your doctor to recommend a nutritionist. They may speed your healing process, through improved nutrition and vitamin therapy.

4. **Enjoy Everyday-**
    - As stroke survivors we recognize the gift we've been given. A stroke can dramatically change your life and that of your family.
    - Keep a gratitude journal. When you hit a rough patch write down all the things you're grateful for. Maybe you're grateful that you shared a laugh with your kids yesterday or you were able to see your grandson hit a homerun or maybe you're grateful for the invention of the cane that guides you around, because life would be tougher without it. It doesn't need to be complicated. Most often when we look at our day we find we're grateful for so many things big and small.
    - Add some comedy to your daily routine. Minimize the drama of the daily news by balancing it with comedy, today's sitcom. How about reruns of "Everybody Loves Raymond?" What's your personal favorite? Study after study has proven the value of laughter in healing.
    - Purchase a joke book and share a few each day- better yet use the library for a constant flow of humorous books.

5. **Effective Emotions-**
    - Negative thoughts and talk lead to negative emotions. Rather than saying-I can't walk – replace it with I am not walking yet. When my vision improves... when my balance improves I am going to... I am not driving yet. My goal is to drive by... always

try to set reasonable goals. Don't allow anyone to limit you.
- Surround yourself with positive, supportive communicators. Example: we enjoyed playing tennis, now we practice tai chi instead. We've put away the sailboat for now and we are learning to play golf together.
- The caregiver needs to monitor the dialog of the family and carefully correct the language used by your loved one.

6. **Enriched Energy-**
    - Every time you accomplish something new, celebrate it, take a breath and set a new goal.
    - Success is in that Plan- the first outings can be tricky. Create a checklist of items needed. For example: medications, water, special food, mobility devices, or oxygen.
    - Make sure to call ahead to inquire about handicap ramps or equipment.
    - Don't try to go to the restaurants at their busiest time.
    - For first outings go on a weekday use reservations or call ahead seating.
    - Avoid weekend entertainment centers; go to the earliest movie maybe during the week.
    - Each time you have a successful travel experience you will be more empowered to try new things. This will prevent feelings of isolation and promote the- "I can do it spirit."

7. **Endurance-**
    - Depending upon your injury, your recovery time can take weeks, months, or years. I have prayed my way through my husband's injuries. As his brain healed it was like he was being reborn. He had to re-learn how to swallow, eat, talk, and walk.
    - For some, managing the recovery can be quite a challenge. Unlike cancer where you might have an oncologist and a family doctor working together or heart disease you might have a cardiologist and a family doctor- my husband's first year healthcare needs required 10 different physician specialists, one family physician and four different therapist. And this was not including his care in the hospital or rehab. This was the care that followed that year or so after.
    - It was an awesome task at times. I had a calendar that kept us organized and also helped at income tax time to gather all the proper receipts.
    - But honestly, the thing that truly helped me through it all was when I decided to take vacations from our worries. We didn't go anywhere but for a few days at a time I refused to think about any problems, no "what ifs." What if this happens or what if that happens. I didn't allow myself to wonder when this would heal or that. The more of these mental vacations that I took the better I coped with the everyday needs of our situation.

- The more I prayed for guidance the more creative energy I found to solve problems.

    The Bible: Matthew 11:28- Come unto me all ye that labor and are heavy laden, and I will give you rest.

8. **Expectation-** *Webster* **definition-**
"The prospect of good to come"
    - That Christmas 2003-It was 5 o'clock in the morning. Chris was now at University of Chicago Neuro Intensive Care Unit. While they rushed to examine him my daughter, my sister, and I sat on a hallway floor waiting for some word, any word. We knew we needed a Miracle for him to survive. We have a large family and we've witnessed numerous Miracles, our fair share joy, but losing another loved one just wouldn't do. I remember pleading with God for another Miracle. I knew the faith and strength of our family and my expectation was that we'd survive this crisis too.
    - We've stopped worrying about what we've lost-we expect that God will work with whatever we have left.

CHAPTER 8
Alpha and Omega

Somewhere in the Journey 2004

People often ask how we're doing. My standard reply is, "we have good days and great days." We've tried to structure our lives in such a way that it's become our truth.

However, there's always that turn in the road. Just when you start to accept a new normal, there might yet be a need for another new normal. Life is full if not complete with change. We've tried to adapt and accept the changes, but there are the in between times, the space in the transition; when you just feel knocked down physically and spiritually. I call them the "dark hole" days.

On this particular dark night sleep finally approached, as the preacher on the religion channel comforted me. When I reached for the remote to turn the television off, the minister's words spoke to me. In a voice set louder than the volume, I heard: "Yes, there is a beginning and an end to all suffering. It... is... Alpha... and Omega he preached a beginning and an end." I knew this wasn't an accident as I drifted into sleep I whispered, "Perfect timing God, thank you."

Did you ever hear just the right words at the absolute right moment? Lying in bed, trying to climb out of the darkness just moments before hearing that minister's voice; my tears were flowing. I literally wanted to scream... I visualized myself imploding in screams.

Through the grace of the minister's voice I was transformed in precious few moments from that "dark hole" to the arms of God. This could only happen when I walked through the pain. How else would I appreciate the good and the great days if never reminded of the dark days?

I wouldn't allow it as often as I should have, but I needed to grieve. I needed to grieve the loss of life that we once knew. I wanted to hear my husband's old voice again. I wanted to see the sparkle in his eyes when he smiled. I wanted to see, and hear his passion again, whether it was about sports or work. We had worked hard, and built a good life together. I wanted to hear him laugh-now he was physically incapable of laughter. He often walked around the house whistling-no more.

My fear was if I focused too much energy on what was missing, I would continue to perpetuate the void. Rather than staying in a state of grace, grateful and positive. It is a tight rope to walk. I should have said okay tonight I'm alone, and I'm going to spend the next two hours grieving what I miss: allow some of these emotions to surface. Instead I would suddenly without warning, and more often in an exhausted state, have this over flow of emotions that I could barely handle.

Then there was my constant companion of guilt. My prayer was that my husband would live, plain, and simple. I placed no conditions of complete health or without suffering, and I promised to work through anything. What about him, for months on end when I watched him suffer, I felt so selfish. "Oh My God," I'd say to myself, "did I really pray for this?"

His brain injury left him with many disabilities. Learning to become more specific, I had a prayer list for…his vision, ability to walk, rebuilding his muscle mass, to eat without a tube, the cognitive issues, mental clarity, paralyzed vocal cords, breathing without the trachea tube, his mind, body, soul and spirit.

Along the way I met many people in the hospital, and rehab waiting rooms. All Angels, I'm sure to this day. They were warm and generous with their feelings. The bonds between us were quick as we shared our loved ones recovery stories. I was amazed to find how many people pray to special Saints. They would often suggest prayers to "Saint…" or pray to Our Lady of … I soon had a prayer list with Saints for every purpose. How's that for specificity? It seemed like an eternity as his body healed, in time both lists were shorter. Was this the beginning of Omega?

Prior to his illness people would often ask me how did we get it all done? We each had full-time careers and he often traveled for work. We had five kids, aging needy parents, and a home. My standard line would be "we divide and conquer". Around holidays or relocations we'd make a list of what we could each manage. I always said that together we had perfect 20/20 vision. He needed glasses for distance and I needed glasses to read. We were a good team and in spite of his illness we still are.

When I needed to be an energy source he could draw from, I had it. When the world couldn't understand him between his tracheotomy and paralyzed vocal cords I could hear him. After a few months of fighting the good fight it became increasing difficult to manage his care, and hold onto my momentum. I had simply allowed myself to get over tired.

I was about to redistribute some responsibilities when my husband prevailed. As his brain healed his mood improved, as did his overall mental clarity. He seemed slightly less selfish, and more engaged in daily life. Finally, more interest in family, what the kids were doing. He was discovering a New Normal. It was now his energy and determination, which carried us through. He woke each day ready to start his daily therapies. His attitude inspired and still inspires me to keep on fighting.

Best Practice:

1. Embrace the pain so you can move through it and past it.
2. It is not only important, but also necessary to give yourself permission to grieve the losses in your life. The act of grieving doesn't make you less grateful for the gifts you been given.
3. Plan your time wisely; it's really not a race.
4. Have your own plan as caregiver for your health and wellbeing.
5. If you have too many "dark days" –seek help it might be depression
6. Forgive yourself for anything you wish you had done differently.
7. Forgive others.
8. You won't create a positive environment if you're angry and upset. Decide what it will take to find happiness in this situation and then set goals to achieve it. You have so much more important work ahead of you.
9. Protect and use your own energy wisely. Find ways to replenish yourself; I would listen to a great preacher on television. Or sit quietly in an old stained glass Cathedral and soak up the peace and spiritual energy. I can sing and dance around to old Motown songs or collapse into a chair enjoying an aria performance from Pavarotti.

CHAPTER 9
Designer Therapies

Late April 2004

When the time was right, I started the process of reassuring Chris that as he healed he would form new connections. "As it was taught to me," I explained, "Think of your brain as a city, with a large infrastructure, highways, bridges and side streets. Some of your bridges are down because of the hemorrhage, however your brain will build pathways around those bridges, and reconnect your thoughts, I promise.

My husband's first love was sports, and still is, he lives and breathes it. Born, and raised in Chicago, he is devoted to all their teams. Even during our twenty year absence, while living on the East Coast, he still found a way through satellite television to follow his beloved Chicago teams.

Three months prior to his suffering a brain hemorrhage he accepted a job transfer for a position in Chicago. Not realizing the significance at the time, it became the perfect catalyst for his impending recovery. When he woke from his coma speaking his first language, Greek, we were back in our birthplace, with his first passion just a channel away. I don't want to mislead you it wasn't magic, "Ta-Dah" the Bulls are on, and he started his rant and rave on the referees as before. No, it happened very gradually.

In the early stages of healing his thoughts weren't clear, and his eyesight was poor. But, this is the guy that as a child would sneak a transistor radio to bed with him at night, to follow the games. Being able to hear the game might have been enough, but viewing even in his limited capacity helped. He received comfort in the familiar, and his natural interest progressed, as his brain was able to focus better. Eventually, the interest turned to enthusiasm, as he planned his therapies around game day schedules.

I knew he had reconnected to his passion, when he threw a box of tissues at the TV, and called The Cubs "a bunch of bums."

All his memories are tied to these teams. He relates to, and categorizes his memories by their accomplishments. For example, in 1996 The Bulls won the championship, and that's the year our oldest granddaughter was born. The Cubs made the playoffs in 2003, we moved that year.

Via sports television he was able to recapture his memories. Those memories transcended him to his early years growing up in the old Chicago neighborhoods. Through the gangways, alleys, and side streets on to the city bus for Chicago Stadium, Wrigley, and Soldiers Field's. As he watched from our living room in his wheelchair, he imagined sitting in the bleachers, smelling the lake air, and feeling the hot humid Chicago summer.

I'm happy to report that he began his process back to us through these old neighborhoods. By stimulating him with his passion, and the familiar, his brain went into construction mode, rebuilding those bridges.

In just a few short months, Chris had grown weary of the repetition of the exercises. To learn how to walk again, his physical therapist had to teach him how to crawl. He hated this. To try to offset some of the hated but important aspects, I tried to search for a way to incorporate some fun. We capitalized on his sports passion and incorporated it into rehab activities. When he had to sing for speech we sang "Take me out to the ball game." We used sports trivia games for memory. We read biographies of his sports heroes. Does your loved one have a special talent, hobby or passion? Can you somehow incorporate it into the daily rehab activities?

Designer Therapies:

1. Always begin your sessions in a safe secure and upbeat environment.
2. Always have your therapies approved by your physician.
3. If you find yourself low on motivation go to your local library to the "self-help" section and take out some books or tapes from motivational speakers. Before you know it you'll be training like Rocky Balboa.
4. When quiet and concentration isn't necessary listen to favorite music or books on tape/disc when exercising.
5. Define what you love-what's your passion?
6. Can you create a realistic program incorporating your passion?
7. Set short term and long term goals for yourself.
8. Write your vision and keep it simple and post it where you'll see it often.
9. Keep a goal plan journal, increasing speed or time. Make it measurable.
10. If vision is a problem, large print books are available from your local library, as are books on tape. Amazon.com also sells used books and tapes. Most computer-generated programs can be viewed in a larger font.

11. While too much TV time is discouraged, used properly it can be an effective tool. Such as, game shows that challenge your mental skills.
12. Could you benefit from an exercise partner? Maybe a neighbor would enjoy a walk.
13. Are you ready for something new and different? Investigate some alternative therapies.
14. Challenge yourself to new levels.
15. Promote healing with Guided Imagery- Bella Ruth Naperstak offers a complete line of products including post stroke help. Her web-site offers tapes/disc on subjects to improve your breathing, visualization techniques or learn to meditate.
16. If you're able to walk try, Tai Chi for relaxation and improved balance.

Best Practice:

1. Design a program that inspires and encourages you. That makes your heart smile and uplifts your spirits.
2. We viewed his recovery as our only fulltime job, it was.
3. He became the customer-I offered him a variety of therapeutic choices.
4. It was structured in a way that his voice leads the way, he had options and choices.
5. He wasn't forced he was encouraged, we made it fun and he got it done.
6. Eventually he took control of planning his own schedule and started to take control of his life.
7. Remember, the longer you can endure your therapy process you will continue to improve.

CHAPTER 10
Prayers and the Specialist

March-June 2004

After prayer, I have my best ideas, I'll wake in the morning with an idea or a solution to a problem. Thankfully, the hospitals all had Chapels, where I often found myself for a few minutes of solitude, and renewal. The Rehab Hospital also employed Pastoral Minister's. They would come to your bedside and pray with you a few times a week. Chris was uncomfortable with this practice. To him prayer is personal.

Baptized Catholic, religion was introduced into my family, though not strictly observed. My parents focused more on teaching us the values of honesty and integrity.

The reverse was true in my husband's family. His grandfather was a Greek Orthodox Priest (Orthodox Priest is allowed to marry.) Chris felt his life was saturated with religion.

My limited exposure kept me desiring more. I searched for and embraced God through prayer. I don't think of myself as very disciplined, although my earliest memories are of me saying my nightly prayers before I went to sleep. A sponge for a sad story, if I heard it that day I prayed for it that night.

Both Baby Boomer's- born of The Depression Era parents, I was often reminded of the luxury that we had simply having food each day, and my parents taught me to appreciate my fortune.

My most perfect prayers were my childhood prayers. Unselfish and pure recited with devotion: "God Bless our family and World let everyone have food to eat, clothes on their back and a smile on their face." I don't recall asking for much for myself. I guess I thought I had it all. Life seemed so simple then. It may have been second hand or leftovers I didn't care. Recounting childhood memories with my younger brother once, he said, "Other kids had chocolate cookies we had vanilla." That probably sums it up best.

My definition of prayer is my on-going dialogue I share with God. My conversations with God sounds something like this-"You know God," I'll say, "I need the best vocal cord doctor in the area." I don't always kneel, sometimes at the kitchen sink doing the dishes; I'll say "you know God I need help with...will you send me an Angel to see me through this."

Before Chris arrived home from rehab I had appointments set-up with three different Ear Nose Throat Doctors- (Otolaryngologist), why three? Because I could, plain and simple, I was going to exhaust all possibilities to aid his recovery. I was determined to find a solution for all of his throat and vocal cord issues. He had already been seen by two doctors that shared the same opinion, I just had a feeling something wasn't right, some piece of his puzzle was missing.

It only took one; he had the same specialty- Otolaryngologist as the others, but a sub specialty in Laryngological studies, and was associated with highly rated Voice Institute. I relayed the same sequence of events to numerous ENT Doctors before him. "He had stroke symptoms, on the way to the ER he aspirated, the emergency tech made numerous frantic attempts trying to intubate him." That's where this specialist stopped me, and said, "Well maybe the cords were injured during the multiple attempts, and they're not paralyzed." He didn't allow me to get too excited, as he went directly to discussing the Vagus nerve, the control center in the cerebellum and the bleed. However under very close examination he felt the vocal cords were indeed scarred together-and Chris was a candidate for surgery. Alleluia-

He was doctor number five.

We saw two Neuro-Ophthalmologists both had the same diagnosis; only one seemed more at ease with him than the other. He was treated with patches, prisms, eye exercises and time.

Talk about a small world. His new Internal Medicine Physician I happened to meet when we brought Chris' mother from Florida to Illinois, and placed her temporarily in an assisted living facility. The doctor had just moved her practice out of Chicago to a suburb near us, and was trying to rebuild her practice. The timing was perfect for Chris, I interviewed her, discussed his needs, and then she guided me on what I missed.

For the two years that he was in her care, she kept her promise to return my calls quickly. She was truly a God send; she examined him once a month, followed all his therapies, and goals. She was my partner in his care, and often said to me that I should write a laypersons guide. We learned so much together. I learned so much from her, and we learned so much from Chris.

By April his "home care" speech therapist told me about a new stimulation device called Vital Stim Therapy. This device can stimulate the paralyzed muscles in his throat that were preventing him from swallowing.

She went on to say it was just approved by the FDA, and there were only a couple of therapists in the Chicago area that have gone through the training, and they already had long waiting lists. I called the company, the individual therapists, and pleaded his case. It's quite a commitment of time when you start the Vital Stim Therapy, its five days a week then four, and decreases gradually. It was an hour's drive each way, and insurance didn't cover it yet, it was expensive but worth it. We started in late May, and within three weeks he was starting to eat small amounts of soft food...Alleluia. Today Vital Stim is covered by most insurance policies.

Best Practices:

1. Most of my research was done on the Internet.
2. Do you have a friend or relative that can help with the time consuming research and help with make the telephone calls?
3. If your insurance company doesn't cover the advanced care or recently approved FDA procedures that should not in any way influence your decision. Example: if they don't cover there must be a reason or they must not need it. An insurance company is just that, don't allow them to make decisions about the care or needs of your loved one.
4. Insurance companies now provide case managers that are able to present your case for authorization for newer products or clinical trials.
5. Don't be confused by the answers to my prayers, God still makes me do the work, sometimes though I think he points me to the right page.
6. Most insurance allows second medical opinions, I took advantage of that.
7. Know the dollar value of your health insurance policy; is it limited in any way? We had good coverage, but it had a cap at one million dollars. If his care went past that we were on our own. Half of the policy was used prior to his coming home. I also had to personally manage his care to achieve its best use financially.

CHAPTER 11
The Birth of New Normals

June 2004-December 2004

It was June and time for Chris' six month check-up post craniotomy. Chris was excited to meet the man that saved his life. Remember he woke from his coma after leaving the hospital.

Though Chris had made significant progress it wasn't progress you could see, it was mostly behavioral and emotional. He was still wheel chair dependent. He spoke only with great difficulty through the trach and paralyzed vocal cords as he thanked him. The doctor studied him as the two men reached out to one another to shake hands.

He is a surgeon, a Neurosurgeon, highly trained, and renowned in his field. But, he was unable to hide his disappointment inside that soft spoken, cool demeanor.

I became painfully aware reading his reactions, that this was not the outcome he had hoped for. When I caught this glimpse of humanity, and genuine emotion, I wanted to hug him.

His first question was, "why did Chris still have the trach?" I explained all the vocal cord, swallow issues, "and until those are resolved I'm told he will need the trach." He said that generally the patient would progress more quickly once the trach is removed. That was certainly something to look forward to. He also reviewed his recent CT scan, and said it showed improvement, his brain was stable.

Even though he could barely speak, Chris wanted to know when he could go back to work. The doctor smiled and rather artfully skirted the question, as he verbally painted this imaginary chart into the air of expectations. "You can expect the majority of recovery by this time frame and then…" he said.

I'd grown weary of these moments, and the possible limiting effect it could have on Chris. The surgery may have been six months prior, but we we're still fully engaged in fighting for his life every day, in every therapy. We were committed to a positive outcome nothing was going to take us off course.

Not sure where the conversation might go…. I politely interrupted. By injecting into the conversation an update on all the therapies we were engaged in. What his daily schedule looked like. The upcoming vocal cord surgery and restorative swallow therapy we had committed to. I asked him if there was anything else we should be doing that I was not aware of.

By directing the conversation, I was in control of the message Chris needed to hear. This often transformed conservation to a more positive tone. The doctor went on to tell Chris about a patient he had seen earlier that day that was still improving four years later. He continued on to say that sometimes the recovery process seems slow. But he wanted us to start comparing month to month, he was sure we find some improvement each time, and we did.

As we were leaving I was sure to make eye contact with him as I held his hand for a moment longer than the handshake and said, "I want you to know I…am…grateful." While I assisted Chris back into his wheelchair, I explained that we were very much in search of our New Normal. He nodded, as though he completely understood. I went on to describe our short term goals, soon he'll be eating again, the trach will be a memory and by the time we come back in six months it will be Christmas and Chris will walk through those doors. He smiled, and said he'd look forward to it.

When I look back at the time Chris was under his care, I can't remember a conversation with him that wasn't truly meaningful. His words were always so carefully chosen. We are not only forever grateful, but have great admiration for him.

June also concluded his home care services. Insurance allowed only ninety days of care. But he could return to outpatient rehab. I made the decision to pay privately for in home care for an additional ninety days. With the time spent in the Vital Stim program, and his impending surgeries I didn't want to take the chance of exposing him to germs back at the rehab center. And Vital Stim was working; he was now in just a four-week period eating soft food. His respiratory infections improved once he came home, as did the aspiration pneumonia. We were fortunate to have some savings.

Late that June, Chris had surgery to repair his scarred together vocal cords. A second surgery followed in August to remove additional granulation that had formed. He had been eating solid food since the end of June. By his September birthday the trach was gone, and they removed his G-tube. That November, he needed a third surgery to close the trach hole, because it didn't heal on its own.

Also that September we tried to do the outpatient rehab. For the sake of history and continuity we scheduled the outpatient services at the rehabilitation hospital; he was in just months before. My memories of his inpatient therapist's were positive, and we looked forward to seeing them. But, what we didn't know is that they were two separate departments. There were no familiar faces when we arrived there.

Day's 1-2-3-Each day we were greeted by a different speech therapist-not acceptable.

Day 3-The physical therapist requested a meeting to tell me he was basically throwing Chris out of therapy. "Chris is too difficult to work with and we should try again in a few months." I did a slow burn just listening to this therapist and I thought, "What the heck, he was never more motivated. He had regained most of his strength. What bring him back when he can walk, and we'll fine-tune his gait? This is crazy, just crazy."

An argument ensued between this therapist and me. He told me Chris was too unsteady and should probably remain wheel chair bound the rest of his life. I couldn't believe what I was hearing.

I was so angry. I don't know what I said to him as I left. Chris however knew something was very wrong, he said, "Please tell me what he said, I saw you yelling at him, and your hands waving, please I need to know," "Why do you care what this idiot said?" I asked. "Because he upset you," Chris replied. "Well he said that you were not ready for more physical therapy, that I should bring you back in a few months after you heal more." Chris replied, "Pam it just doesn't matter what they say or think we know the truth." As it was our custom then, because of his speech impediments, I then repeated everything he said back to him to be sure I understood him. And then I added, "You're so right Honey, I know you are," as I took a deep slow breath.

Day 4-I forced a meeting with one of their Rehab- Doctors/Physiatrist and she remembered Chris, as she had filled in for his previous doctor many times. She examined him and questioned him. She felt that he had made great progress and was impressed with his attitude. She over-rode the therapist decision and said he was to start back with a new physical therapist, the next morning. I waited as I requested she put her decision in writing.

Day 5-I called their administrator and fired them. Why did I bother to wait the day before for that report? Therapists have the ability to prevent your continued therapy. If you're not motivated or having other health difficulties they can put your therapies on hold. I wasn't going to allow this to happen for Chris.

I found a rehabilitation company for his physical therapy near the house. He started with them that same week of September and was taking steps by mid December.

Christmas 2004- It happened exactly the way I predicted that June day in the Neurosurgeon's office. He proudly walked in for his one-year check up, through those doors, with a cane and no tubes attached to his body. There was one exception, the Doctor was attending to an emergency patient and missed it. We understood, but were very disappointed.

Later that week Chris had more opportunities to show off, and he did. While he wasn't ready to give up his wheelchair completely, as our kids arrived home for the Christmas Holiday their Dad walked to the doorway to greet them. Their marred memories of a Christmas past, flying to us in that traumatic state, were replaced in one year with tears of joy, their Dad the "Miracle Man." Let this "Christmas 2004", be the one that they remember most.

Best Practices:

1. Studies have shown written goals are more often achieved than verbal goals.
2. Celebrate each achievement no matter how small.
3. Praise your loved ones efforts often they need constant reinforcement.
4. You do have options; you don't have to accept inadequate care.
5. Remain open to new ideas and alternative therapies.
6. If a therapist or doctor is not a positive influence, I would cut ties and hire a new one.
7. During the interview process if I couldn't establish a comfortable relationship with that person I kept looking. He's welfare in that fragile state had to be protected.
8. There was one question I often asked of the medical professionals that were involved in my husband's care-What would you do f this were your loved one? How would you handle this? It took their thoughts to a more personal level, and I believe those questions provided us the best possible and honest responses.

CHAPTER 12
The Paradox-Phenomenon-Plateaus

Reflection of 2004

Nothing appeared to come to us easy, each step was a battle. Although, according to some we were accomplishing the impossible, and our results that year were amazing. This made the struggle worth it.

Beginning with the absolute peace, and gratitude I felt watching him, with those first swallows of food. The sense of pride the day that trach came out, the relief when the G-tube was removed, or the joy in those first steps. It was only a few steps at first, he only needed one, and the rest would come.

It was a year poised in Paradox-The very same system that fought to save his life would seriously underestimate his future potential. These were the experts. Remember the doctor that said he might never be without the trach or G-tube or the therapist that said he would never walk again. Or how about the doctor that was ready to perform urinary tract surgery, because some brain injury patients need it. Chris only needed more water.

Did they not understand the extraordinary power they had over these fragile brains they were caring for, the damaging effects. How their suggestion could have devastating limiting consequences. There were times when I wished I could put a filter on them. Thank God, Chris and I are wired differently, you tell us we can't and we'll show you how.

With the best of intentions they would warn, "Well you know typically this that or the other has healed by now." His "home service" physical therapist told me at about six months post surgery that Chris' core (abdomen) should be stronger by now, with less Ataxia. I had great respect for her; she worked so hard with Chris, and truly like so many others seemed to care about him. I listened carefully, and studied what she said. My first question was, "is that six months after surgery or six months after they're awaken from their Coma?" Certainly the patient that's been in a coma for three of those months shouldn't be held to the same standard. My second question was, "did the patients that had the full six months to strengthen their core have a G-tube protruding from it?"

I had great respect, and admiration for most of his doctors and therapists, but we didn't always agree.

At the end of the day it didn't matter to me who was right or wrong, my message was clear we're not done fighting. If you weren't a positive influence in his recovery, I made the change in a heartbeat.

Here in lies the paradox in Neurology. When you ask for a time frame of the healing processes after brain injury, your told that every brain is different they heal differently, and regrettably that's all the information they can give you.

However, when healing doesn't begin, and end within a specific time frame, alarms go off. Because, it appears the medical community does have some guidelines or a system of measurement that it uses. You need to take into consideration the obvious before you over react. When they say the core should be healed in six months, did they plan to have a large plastic cap, and cord hanging from it? Well no, I don't think so, revert to their original advice, and don't panic. "We all heal differently."

Over this course of time, I found we simply exhausted the expertise of a particular doctor or therapists. No one's at fault it just happens. It was time for a change or new eyes on his care to take him to the next level.

My husband is often greeted by a doctor after reviewing his file with a handshake and words like, "You know you're supposed to be dead don't you?" Or "Do you know how rare it is to live through a brain hemorrhage this size?" My personal favorite "Do you know what a gift you've been given?" Soon led me to start the process of documenting my husband's illness, and survival, because I understood our Miracle came with a purpose. Also, I didn't forget my promise that Christmas Night.

The Bible; Luke 12:48-"To whom much is given much is required."

But, I would wonder about those comments that were made by his doctors, "You know you should be dead," and often ask myself how Chris was being measured? Against what- If only a few survive a brain hemorrhage of this size, is it those few he's compared with, who knows those few? I soon came to realize we were writing the script for those rare survivors, many of the rules didn't apply. No one really knew the extent of the brain damage he incurred that night, waiting all those hours for care. The doctors and therapists I respected most would tell me they didn't know for sure, "but let's try this based on these symptoms."

Having said all that, sometimes it's not the doctor or course of treatment, it's the patient, and they simply plateau. Chris has had many plateaus throughout the years. But, we hang on to our hope, and the words of his Neurosurgeon when he said to look for any improvement, though small it maybe. We also needed a more reasonable system of measurement as time went by, we didn't check or evaluate his progress month to month anymore, and change didn't come as quickly. Often by comparison we were able to see improvement over a six-month period or huge improvements from year to year.

From a stable period of healing and renewal, is when a plateau or regression was so painfully obvious. Immediately I was on the phone to his doctor's office, frightened by his symptoms, "he seems so off, his eye sight, speech, mental clarity, and his balance." Well, his doctors humored me the first few times with a CT scan or a MRI. Thankfully, they always found the brain was healing well, and was stable. I still didn't have an answer as to why this is happening.

After experiencing a few of these episodes, I recognized a pattern developing. The phenomenon is, he will struggle with these symptoms for seven to ten days at a time but, always comes out of it with a new-found ability or clarity. Today almost five-year post craniotomy, he still goes through these periods of rebuilding. Again, when I ask no one seems to know why.

As recently as last week, I had the opportunity to ask this question. He was the speaker for our stroke group, an Internist that specialized in strokes. I explained to him this phenomenon and asked if he had any knowledge of this. He didn't other than to say that Neurologist once thought that all healing from stroke/brain injury happened in the first year or two. They now know, the healing continues for years.

Chris' life continues to teach us about the healing brain, and sometimes defies logic. Just as it did the night we prayed for a Miracle. At that point his death was scientifically logical, his life defies it.

Best Practices:

1. No one can protect the information flow, to your loved one, as the caregiver can. Direct the message and protect their environment.
2. Everyone comes up against a wall or a plateau during a long illness; try to employ positive methods to pull out of it. Ask doctors and therapists for help.
3. Sometimes change in routine will help. Sometimes just taking a short break from the routine will help.
4. I found a great motivator is gratitude-to me it's a "State of Grace."
5. During a plateau make lists of what you're grateful for.
6. We make travel lists of places we want to visit. We try to transform the mundane.
7. Don't assume it is plateaus; always get the advice of your doctor.

CHAPTER 13
All You Need Is Love

Yesterday, Today & Tomorrows

People looked at Chris after his brain injury, and saw a man that made them uncomfortable. They would often and quickly turn away.

I witnessed our grandchildren's eyes, and how they didn't miss a step when greeting him. They rushed to his arms unaffected by the tubes, they saw only the good- they saw him.

Our sons had become men and hand shaker's, however their expression of affection changed with their Dad's illness. From the beginning of Chris' illness they each took turns, and came for a weekend to help out. In the morning they would find him up waiting for them in his wheelchair-I sat amazed; as I would watch our big guys gently embrace their Dad. Each of our sons greeted him with their arms around his shoulders, and a kiss on the top of his head. How did they each know what to do? I was so proud of them.

Our daughters are more easily affectionate. They didn't leave or arrive home, without hugs and kisses, and "I love you Dad." Their love and commitment runs deep. They literally put their life outside of work on hold for his needs, and my need for a break. I experienced the best of my family in the worst of times.

I saw his heart, that was still beating for me, I felt his spirit though more fragile, I embraced my husband, a man in need of healing.

Is the prescription love? This illness will test your love as it tests your faith. You'll search through your loved ones injuries trying desperately to find them somewhere in the aftermath. Yes love, we write beautiful songs and stories about it. It sounds so easy, though realistically to achieve this can be difficult. To react to someone in a loving manner, when their actions are rather unlovable, and his or her words aren't beautiful, is your toughest test.

Our marriage united my two sons from a first marriage, and two children (son & daughter) from my husband's first marriage. Only days before we would celebrate our first wedding anniversary, our baby girl made five. The second year of marriage was celebrated with my husband receiving sole custody of his children. This was in the early 1980's. The details of his grant for sole custody had to be extraordinary, and they were. Needless to say, his kids then ages 5 and 3 ½ were in need of special help, and would be for years to come. We were well prepared by the mental health community for possible problems they would encounter as they worked through the events of their early childhood. Not ready to accept this dark future they were painting for the kids I simply asked, "So how do I help them now?" One of the more senior psychologists in this group spoke up and said, "Take them home and love them, just love them. That is what they need the most."

My younger sister died suddenly from a heart attack. She was only 41 years old. She left behind three young children ages 7, 9 and 11. We were devastated by her loss. She was needed by so many. It made no sense, she was too young. She appeared to be the vision of health, and beauty as she was presented in her casket.

I can remember walking the grounds of the funeral home that night mentally preparing her eulogy for the next morning when a family friend found me. He walked patiently for a while with me, and made the appropriate small talk. It took me a while to really open up my heart that night but, I began, and as I said the words, "her children" I began to cry.

He too had lost his mother at a young age, and would only agree that their lives would be difficult for a while. But, he insisted the kids will be well cared for and that "they'll get through it. Just love them, that is what they really need, love them." Anyone else might have been kicked to the curb that night to suggest that we would ever be all right without her.

Oh, and don't forget Bernadette his nurse from rehab, of course when he was being discharged it was her advice that I pursued. "Take him home and love him. Love him every day," she advised.

Our oldest grandson Shane is now 14. When I ask about his future he assures me that he is going to live this awesome and cool life as a Skateboard Dude. Just what every grandparent wants to hear. It sounds happy, I guess. With this chosen profession you must have long hair. I disagree with the length, he looks messy. I suggested leaving it a little longer but maybe styled differently. I offer all my wisdom on the hair issue: how important your appearance is and I could go on for quite a while, but I won't. On this day Shane had planned to spend the night. Prior to his Dad leaving he warned Shane "you know your Nana probably won't give up on you- getting a haircut. Are you sure you don't want to come home?" Shane replied, "Dad don't worry I can handle Nana! Go home!" No one realized I could hear them.

The next morning at breakfast I looked at my grandson across the table from me and said, "I overheard you and your Dad yesterday. Yes... I believe your words were," "Dad don't worry I can handle Nana"...so is this true that you think you can handle me?" Shane smiled looked directly into my eyes and said, "That's true Nana because I happen to know you love me more than you hate my hair." Oh how right he is.

Is love the prescription, I believe so, and hopefully you have it in an unconditional abundance.

The mood imbalance associated with brain injury can be quite cruel. I remind you that it is the injury; it's not your loved one. You too must remind yourself of that, as you experience these possible personality changes, it's only temporary.

Some days you might need a thicker skin. Wear it and try to remember a happier time; a loving moment, a special experience you shared together. Do whatever you need to do to get through this process with limited reaction. Know the brain will heal, and you will have less regrets having loved them through it.

Best Practices:

1. Love them more on the days that they are unlovable; they are trying to fight their way back to you
2. Remind them daily that they are loved-it helps give purpose to the battle.
3. Even the acceptance of affection may be difficult at first for some survivors of stroke/brain injury. It may be over stimulating.
4. Arguments should be avoided, re-focus their attention to something more positive.
5. Don't take the rejection personally-it all about a healing brain. It's about the patient.
6. Chris felt safest in his wheelchair, for months on end he refused to sit on the sofa next to me; he said it made him feel anxious. Respect their needs and remind yourself, it's temporary.
7. Reassurance is so important. The injury can make them feel vulnerable and insecure in a relationship that they once felt secure in.
8. Love will make the difference.

CHAPTER 14
New Year- New Goals

One Year Post Craniotomy- 2005

That January began on a positive note when I was able to send back all the respiratory equipment, oxygen and the wheelchair. Once they removed the equipment I rushed to clean the areas where it was stored. I moved the furniture to replace the void of the wheelchair. I wanted it gone, the memory, and the purpose it once served out of my home. It was as though to not turn that page as quickly as possible, I'd be inviting trouble.

After a celebration of the year one accomplishments it was time to address the rest of the list. While so much healing occurred first year, pushed and prodded by wonderful specialists, we still had a multiple of disabilities to contend with. It was time to set our goals for the New Year.

Chris has two eye conditions as a result of the injury, diploma (double vision) and nystagmus. In addition to his prisms and large font reading exercises, it was recommended he started using video games for hand/eye coordination. It was a fun addition to his daily therapies.

His walk is still unsteady and ataxic; he walks like he's drunk. To hear him describe it he doesn't walk across a room without a plan. He would probably be steadier if he would use a cane. But he refuses to, claiming he never falls, and he doesn't want to be dependent on it. His physical therapy sessions and his daily exercise routine that he created are ongoing. We became mall walkers three mornings a week. It broke up some of the monotony of winter.

Once he recovered from the profound dysphasia and had the trach removed the speech problems were still severe. His diagnosis is- dysthrasia and reclaiming his speech has been the toughest task. We spent his first year in speech therapy with focus on swallow techniques and rebuilding flexibility to his vocal cords. Our focus year two was to begin to rebuild his speech and voice. We found a wonderful, experienced speech therapist in private practice. His goal for year two was to be understood. He wanted to order food in restaurants, talk to our kids on the phone and be less dependent on me to be his voice.

One of the largest roles I played during his recovery was that of his speech therapy/aide. Each day, as natural as brushing our teeth, making the bed or having breakfast we worked on his speech. This practice began as he woke from his coma and the therapies started. I have worked with him on his speech at least five days a week. In the beginning in rehab he was scheduled for two-thirty minutes sessions daily. At night I would do a-twenty-minute reinforcement. When in home therapy came three days a week, I filled in the rest of the week with two half-hour sessions daily and as his attention span returned at minimum an hour a day. We work on his speech to this day.

The plan is always under the guidance of a speech therapist. But I did try to create sessions that are either more fun or more challenging. In conjunction with speech therapy, I focused my efforts on rebuilding his vocabulary. We often spent more time on the four or five syllable words. I would use a dictionary to reintroduce words common to his prior vocabulary always a reinforcement of the reconnection process or awakening using the familiar. Because speech was so difficult for him it was hard to measure his verbal thoughts or abilities. So we used a business dictionary and once he was able to say the word or business term; I started to test him on defining them. He knew the answers. I suggested a project where he develops a business model or concept, and develop a marketing plan for it. As I defined it for his therapist he had two levels in his writing that he used. The first was similar to how he expressed himself prior to injury. The second was how he needed to express himself since the injury. Post injury he would shorten his sentences to over articulate the words to be understood. His first real attempt of a writing project he seemed to move back and forth between the two levels. Some sentences were beautifully articulated, while others were chopped up as he did for ease of speech. So was the language center intact and being affected by his inability produce clear speech? Or was he rebuilding the language center and some aspects were still in process. Either way the goal was to continue to build the language center and eliminate the choppy speech.

Another goal for year two, he wants to drive. After the approvals of all doctors involved we started the driving process. We went to parking lot of a closed warehouse and practiced every day. It took about a year before he felt safe enough to drive alone. He went only a short distance a mile or more, early afternoon, with perfect weather conditions and in light traffic.

A hard but good year, his daily therapies were all consuming. As the 2005 Fall Harvest came in, Chris too started to reap the rewards of his efforts. He could speak well enough to be understood, which gave him the confidence and independence to try to venture out to the store alone. He started to drive at the same time his Mom went into a nursing home. She fell again, and broke her other leg. He had a cell phone for emergencies. I still worried whenever he went out the door. I was grateful to have his help with visits to his Mom though. He now had confidence, some independence and he was needed, he had a purpose, taking care of his Mom.

As he healed, grew stronger and accomplished more each day, he also had a revelation of acceptance. He told me, "you know when I sit in this chair I feel like I can do anything, but then I get up." He also accepted he was not ready to return to the type of upper level management positions he once enjoyed. "Not yet," he said, "and maybe I'll have to create a different future for myself." Maybe this was an easier place for him to get to and accept once he began to achieve other milestones. I was just so relieved we got there. It allowed me the opportunity to discuss with him a more realistic future. I was committed to not strip him of his hope of returning to work. It was one of his greatest motivators. This was another prayer answered.

With the job issue out of the way; I could now approach the subject of selling that huge house that we could no longer afford and moving back to the East Coast to reunite our family- children and grandchildren. Chris' recovery was very rewarding, but I needed my joy back-my family. By the New Year 2006, I had the house ready to sell.

Best Practices:

1. When possible allow your loved one to come to terms or acceptance with their limitations due to injury, in their own time frame.
2. Remember if something is currently an unattainable goal, it may very well be achieved at a later date.
3. Keep hope alive as Chris did when he said he might have to create his own future.
4. Devise an action plan to create future opportunities relative to their abilities.
5. Maybe what was once a hobby or a passion could become a source of income with some imagination.

CHAPTER 15
Saying Good-Bye

New Year 2006

I was excited about spending more time again with our grandchildren. I had visions of jumping in a mud puddle with our grandsons, getting dirty, daughter in laws furious, and giggling about it, with my little guys. Just stirring up trouble, I'm such a rebel. Life had been so serious I just longed to play. I wanted to cook a nice meal for my big family, with my granddaughters helping in the kitchen, chopping away, singing to Aretha Franklin or Patti LaBelle. Children are running everywhere. I needed to hear babies crying, children laughing, our kids disagreeing on everything and anything- I needed my organized chaos back.

When we we're saying our good-byes to the Neuro Ophthalmologists that followed Chris' care for those two years, she expressed her gratitude to Chris for teaching her "that people do heal." She said she really didn't expect to see his recovery. I was so surprised. I told her that I never expected to hear this from her, she was always so supportive. Then I joked that I would never ever play poker with her. Boy, did I read her wrong. I realized how difficult saying that was for her, as she appeared to tear up. I said, "Well, I guess the two of you were meant to meet and have this chapter together." She replied, "Yes, isn't God great." "Indeed He is," I replied, "Indeed He is."

We had similar discussions as we said our good-byes to all his doctors/therapists that we had handpicked for his recovery, what an awesome team. We shared mutual respect, admiration and best wishes. He had come so far, he became the pride of his therapists.

Chris' life and injury has touched the lives of so many.

The hardest part for me was saying goodbye to my Mom. When she saw that my daughters were able to take care of Chris for short periods, my Mom forced me away from him. We spent a couple of hours on Sunday afternoons together for lunch and shopping. She's brilliant; it was the best medicine for both of us. It was almost cruel that after so many years we would have this opportunity to spend more time together and need to part again. Mom is rooted there, and I am meant to be near my kids, I just can't have it all.

When Chris was in the hospital, my oldest sister (our nurse) devoted endless days to Chris' care. She also guided me through his process. Our family is very fortunate to have her. As in the past, she is beyond generous with her time, to our family need or crisis.

I'm grateful as well to my younger brother, Chris' buddy, who often dropped in for sports talk, and an iced tea.

Then we have our family's comic relief, another older sister, always finds the humor in our tragedies. Oh, how we needed to laugh.

Today, and better than ever, I am able to see God's perfectly orchestrated plan....

From that moment in 2003 when discussions came up about this promotion/move, I was so resistant. For so many years, I was supportive of Chris' success. But, I never had to leave our kids before. The harder I resisted, the more the Chicago move fell into place. The final promise was he would be traveling less. And the way he said he was tired, and tired too of the travel, my alarm went off. He had never complained before. I immediately surrendered to the move.

When I hired the realtor to purchase the Chicago area house my specifications were simple, "I want a nice house in an area where I can resell it quickly." I already had the exit strategy in place. The house I chose had a very modern kitchen, with a large counter that sat eight. It was attached to a large, open family room, with huge windows overlooking a lake. With a first floor master suite that over looked the lake as well. The realtor cautioned me about the kitchen, he thought it might be too modern for some wanting the traditional kitchen table. "The house might not sell as quickly," he warned. I didn't care. I wanted that house. I thought I was buying it for me until he had the stroke.

Do you know that counter became his parallel bars, which were used for him to walk again?

The fact that I had the first floor master allowed me to take him home early.

The lake was a perfect backdrop for the healing environment for him and me. I looked out the window every day, and said, "Thank you God for this beautiful view."

If -his Mom hadn't fallen when she did, there was no reason for us not to stay another day in Maryland. Because, we wouldn't leave her alone, we traveled home Christmas Day, and spent that evening with her.

If the airline didn't lose our luggage we would have gone to bed sooner. The luggage arrived thirty minutes before the paramedics were called.

We kept his Angels very busy that Christmas Night. Chris had an appointment with his destiny. His Neurosurgeon left hours after performing Chris' surgery for a vacation. We only had a short window available for his services. And I know now... it had to be him.

My youngest daughter said to me one night when we were living in Maryland, "Mommy those people talk like you." We were watching the Chicago News; I smiled at the thought of maintaining my Chicago accent after all those years.

There's something to be said about the familiar, hearing the voices of people in the grocery stores that sound just like you is comforting.

To be home for both of us under those extraordinary circumstances was another blessing. He had his Chicago Sports TV. This is how he learned to speak English as a child; only Greek was spoken in his home.

I had the comfort of my family, my Mom, sisters and brother for additional support. You don't need to entertain them. You can all sit silently together and still be heard, their family.

Even though I missed our sons terribly, I think it was best for me not to have my focus spilt in any way, Chris had all my attention.

Our every need was met indeed; it was a perfectly orchestrated plan.

Best Practices:

1. Best lessons are realized during a reflective period when you can see the beauty or the purpose in the transformation.
2. Accept your fate graciously it's your wisdom and character builder.
3. Understand that your life may be used as an example, for the greater good.
4. Try to find time to jump in a mud puddle-
5. Make a snow Angel-
6. Take a walk in a warm soft rain.
7. Cherish and protect your family, they are your best assets.

CHAPTER 16
The Goal: "The Speech"

March 2006-We landed in Hanover PA.

With that solid exit strategy, I sold that house in record time in a housing market that was just starting to turn, it was time to go. I was being released from my surrender two years before. Our daughter in law inspected houses for me that I would find on the Internet. She also chose the nursing home for Chris' mother. I flew in for a day inspected our picks and submitted a contract. I then flew back to Chris that night. Our sons rented a couple of trucks packed us up and took us home. Not like the old days when Chris' company would send professional movers. Boy, did I miss that service.

My goal was to be within an hour radius of our three son's homes. I chose a town that borders Maryland and Pennsylvania to achieve this. The town itself had to meet certain criteria: I wanted the advantages of a larger town in a country setting with: public transportation, shopping, movie theaters, a good nearby General Hospital and ample medical services.

I have shared with our kids since Chris' illness how my priorities have changed. "My goal is to live at least one day longer than your Dad." Because, my family has not been blessed with longevity as has his-I'm forced to think about these things. I don't dwell on them although I have tried to prepare accordingly. I want him to have ease in everyday living and all advantages if he should ever be alone.

Moving for us really isn't the stressful event that most endure, we seek a new adventure. We have a large oil painting of Chris' grandfather the Greek Orthodox Priest, I mentioned earlier. We carefully have this family treasure crated when we move and it's the first thing we unpack and hang to prevent any destruction to it. Over the years our kids have claimed his eyes in the painting follow them, my usual reply is, "there must be something you feel guilty about. Do you want to talk about it?" Out of habit and respect we hang it in a place of prominence, and say "We're home." It's almost that quick for us.

We celebrated my birthday about a week after we moved into the new house. I received the best present that year when my husband wrote me a letter expressing his feelings and gratitude. With great clarity and a familiar tone, he was present in it. I heard his old voice, and his thoughts, being expressed through the writing. There was even some humor. He said, "If you could have found a way for my teams to win all the time, you would have." He was absolutely correct; nothing would have made me happier.

We came full circle that year with our gift giving. In our early years of marriage we couldn't afford gifts for each other, so we just took care of our kids. This practice always bothered Chris more than it did me. He promised the day would come when he would make it up to me. He did so, for many years, with extravagant gifts. But, that letter brought me peace on so many levels. We turned another corner.

This year Chris really started to take more control over his destiny. He had more rules for me however; I was allowed to only participate in his first doctor/ therapy appointments to help shed light on his history. Any future appointments he wanted to go alone. I agreed, with one suggestion, "during my visit, goals were to be established. They should be your goals, I added, but I want to make sure I understand the strategy going forward." Everything seemed to be up for negotiation for awhile as he took charge of his life.

We were fortunate to find great doctors and therapist all within two miles of our new home.

His mother has received last rites four times in recent years. She spent a year in Hospice until they could no longer justify it; she recovered again, another mystery in my life. Her nursing home is a mile away, and Chris visits her every other day.

Being surrounded by family again was the best thing for him. While we couldn't fill the hours in the day with a dream job yet, our grandchildren provided numerous time consuming possibilities. We have school concerts, award ceremonies, grandparent's days, and the entire field of sports-softball- soccer-football-basketball, yes they are his grandchildren. Having our sons nearby to share a beer and watch a ball game is awesome.

A few months after our move Chris described to me an awakening of sorts that was happening to him; he described it as "everything seems so much clearer to me now," Alleluia.

Chris has been blessed with many natural gifts; one is a talent for public speaking. Other speakers would dread following him after his speech, he was always a tough act to follow.

His speech goal that year was to speak publicly again. While, I felt it was slightly ambitious, I supported him. He really enjoyed working with his new speech therapist. She is young, energetic, supportive and determined to help him achieve his goals. We just adore her.

About one year after setting the public speaking goal he had his speech written, almost completely memorized and now an audience. In conjunction with our local hospital a stroke support group was formed.

My heart was pounding as he began his speech. When he got through his first line, and I heard their laughter, I was soon at ease. They were able to understand him and his joke. My God, he did it. I was so proud of him.

It's true, he is still a tough act to follow even through his strained speech he connects with, and inspires his audience. I followed him with a speech on caregivers, and spoke about one of my favorite topics- him.

Here are short excerpts from his speech.

Surviving a Brain Injury-By Chris Papas
For the stroke support group-
May 9, 2007

I started as a regular guy. I have a wonderful wife and raised five kids. Now I'm a grandfather six times. And if I knew how good that was going to be, I would have skipped parenthood and gone straight to being a grandfather.

I was successful in my career, which was the restaurant and hotel business. I created, or played a part in several national brands. I was the C.O.O./President of the largest company owned hotel group in the country. But I was not ready for what was about to happen to me.

I spent Christmas 2003 with my family at my son's house in Maryland. Upon flying back to Chicago, Christmas Day, I got a headache as we were getting ready for bed. I don't re-

member anything for the next five weeks, but I was told that I was taken for brain surgery. I was in a coma for five weeks.

You'll find yourself getting stronger and smarter each day. Even when you don't realize it, if you're doing what you're supposed to, you'll get better. As was stated you would find yourself being afraid of a lot of things, especially new things. This is good. It lets you know that you are about to do something that will take extra care. However, you cannot avoid doing everything that you are afraid of. If that were the case you would never try anything. When you do try something and fail at it. It is not the end of the world. Just pick yourself up and try again. You'll find that the more you do something, or try to do it, the better at it you become.

At first you will only want to do things that you are comfortable with. There is a saying that today is the first day of the rest of your life. Well, that is very true in your situation. And what you do today will have a great bearing on what you are tomorrow. Nothing happens right away, but nothing can happen without an effort from you. You can be whatever you want to be. The future is in your hands.

He mesmerized the crowd for about a half an hour. He had note cards, in large print that he rarely had to refer to. He did get off track a couple of times, but regrouped without notice. He never got nervous even when he lost his place, he didn't lose he confidence. I've heard his presentations many times throughout the years, and as before if he went off track he found his way back. He is a natural public speaker. Later he said, "You know, I think we're a pretty interesting hour."

We were asked to speak again. Chris wrote and presented a second speech six months later. This speech is an improvement over the previous speech six months earlier, some more excerpts:

Designer Therapies:
The Speech for Stroke Group
November 13, 2007

As we grew up the world continued to change around us, however to borrow a quote from the movie Field of Dreams, - "the one constant was baseball" and I loved it.

My Dad came to this country at 12 years old, a Greek immigrant; he worked all his life to make things better for others. I remember growing up and the whole family would be around the dinner table. It didn't matter what time it was, we always waited for Dad to have dinner. Anyway I remember sitting there in Chicago, where I grew up, and my Dad would ask me why I cared what the Cubs did that day. "Will they care about you when your bills are due? Will they wonder what you did when you get older?"

I did not know how to explain to him that it did not matter to me if they cared or not. I knew I cared about what they did. Soon my attention was drawn by lots of different sports. In the fall it was football, in the winter there was hockey, and starting in 1966 basketball. The spring and summer had baseball; for me the Cubs and the Sox. I remember reading sports books by the hall light and keeping a transistor radio under my pillow just to listen to the ball game that night. I was always drawn to this. My parents could never understand it, but I didn't care. It was important to me and I've never lost my passion for sports.

After the craniotomy things were never the same. However, one thing I could always relate to is what was happening in sports. The scores made sense. The years of research and reading I had done made following the story lines doable for me. Something that involved sports was more interesting and more logical to me.

Another thing that I understood was the daily training sessions I had to go through. If I was going to get better, like I planned, I had to work at it every day. I knew this and I accepted it. But, that didn't mean that I didn't hate doing it. I would go through the routine prescribed for me by the Doctors and therapists. Every day I would do the same thing to make myself better, boring as it was. And it was, until Pam came up with a way to make it more interesting.

Chris' Favorite Quote-

When I don't want to do what I know I should, I look at a stone cutter hammering away perhaps a hundred times without making the slightest crack. Yet on the hundred and first blow it will split in two. I know it was not that blow that split the stone but all that went before it...

Author Unknown

That year Chris gave three wonderful speeches and was even a guest speaker on an area talk radio show with his therapist. Dreams came true in 2007.

Best Practices:

1. Never, Never Give Up
2. It doesn't need to be perfect you just need to try.
3. You need to know when to let go. He was ready to fly before I was ready for him to leave the nest.
4. Surround yourself with people that support your goals. He achieved much more with a therapist when their goals were aligned.
5. Let your loved one know when you're proud of them- Chris told me later that it wasn't about the speech he wanted his family to be proud of him again.
6. If I knew then, what I know now, I wouldn't have worried so much.
7. Try to find joy, peace and acceptance in each day.
8. Constant encouragement and reassurance is needed to get through this process.

CHAPTER 17
The Editor

Winter 2008

I am a truly fortunate person. My life has been rich with abundance. My blessings began the day I was born the "middle child" into a large family, often the bridge between the older and the younger siblings. We didn't always understand each other, but we always treasured each other.

Our marriage was challenged from the beginning, when we blended our broken families together. Today, you could never guess which child had blood ties; they belong to each other and us. As each of our five children struggled growing up they taught me to love deeper and pray more.

My husband and I are opposites. But, we have always respected and embraced our differences. We are friends. Though he often felt I was complicated, he'd say, "You operate from an extra sense that I just don't have." At the same time, I was always in awe of him because he was so darn smart. He seemed to know everything I didn't know. It was those differences that forced our growth as people.

With the many titles I've owned in my life and hats I've worn, I found my greatest gift is being his wife; the love we share and of our family. I have discovered a new depth to our family and the love that unites us. When one of is hurt, we all hurt. In my heart we are one, "one love," as we are all spiritually connected.

Adding the Caregiver title to my list of achievements holds some my most heartfelt thoughts, soulful feelings and cherished memories. I no longer question its purpose in my life. Through writing this book I have satisfied my need of finding joy "in the moment." I have realized that for me, my true joy is in giving.

The *Thesaurus*' definition of *Joy* is fun. To me and to my life joy and fun are very different. Joy is felt in my soul and fun is an emotion of my spirit. My expectation is when we're up on that hilltop dancing we're going to have some fun.

A lifetime of lesson learned and each coping skill I have mastered was utilized during this period of time. I have never worked so hard mentally or physically. Nor have I ever dug so deep into my own soul for survival.

Last winter Chris said, "I'm going to write something just for me, just for fun." I encouraged him and said, "Go for it." Before I knew it he was writing a sports book.

By Spring I was editing. Line by line, I was engaged not only in his gift of writing, but how he used his passion to develop his craft, and to heal his wounds.

Somewhere inside of Chris is a sports announcer bottled up and ready to call the "play-by-play." In the meantime, or until he's discovered by ESPN, he expresses his passion in his recently copyrighted book.

"Three Strikes"
Author: Chris Papas
Here's an excerpt-

"Ball one," cried the umpire. The next pitch Nick threw was supposed to be around the knees but was around the ankles. "Ball two" bellowed the Ump. Now Nick was behind two balls to one strike and Mountain had not even swung his bat. Nick knew that the next pitch had to be a strike. Mountain knew it too. Nick decided he was going to rear back and fire one. Whatever was going to happen was going to happen. Nick wound up and threw one as hard as he could to where Vince was expecting it. Vince saw the ball coming and set his glove to catch it. The ball never got there. Mountain saw the ball too. He swung with all of his might, making sure that he would hit the ball. The pitch Nick threw was turned around quickly, going on a plane toward center field. Speed turned around as soon as he heard the crack of the bat. He knew this was going to be well hit and going a long way. He turned and raced to the fence, talking to the ball the whole time- "Sink you devil sink." But the ball didn't sink. Instead it got even higher as it passed over the fence where Speed was headed. Speed and Nick looked like a matched pair; both with their hands resting on their knees and breathing like they had just run a marathon. That hit knocked all the wind out of them and they watched the two Central runners round the bases. They knew that this would put them behind by one in what might have been the most important game they had played up to that point.

He was filled with enthusiasm as he wrote "Three Strikes." It was such a pleasure to experience this with him.

Although, he's not the picture of health yet, he is the positive example of what life can be; for those that survive and conquer the devastation of stroke/brain injury.

So now I'm his Editor, another title, I never would have imagined. I'm so proud of him; he can still render me speechless.

Remember, it was me… when I said "I'm not much for mysteries, I will stop and ask for directions if I'm lost. I don't like to waste time." While all the above is still true, a more patient me understands that I may have to be still, and wait for an answer.

Although, sometimes frustrated by the unknowns of his injury, I try to stay focused on the end result. I don't know yet exactly what it will look like; Chris is still healing. But, none the less, I remain dedicated to the best possible outcome.

For the purpose of developing this Caregiver's Guide, one of my intentions was to address the need of taking time to mentally prepare you for the journey ahead. I can only express and encourage the importance, now knowing, the difference it will make. Your attitude and emotional health will set the tone, and become the fabric of the healing environment that you create for your loved one. Finally, I'll remind you, your endurance is the key.

"Reclaiming a Life of Significance," is much more than just carefully chosen words. It was and remains our mission. We set new goals each year to manage the chronic ailments that were the result of the brain injury. We are flexible and understand better than ever, that life will bring changes. We may have to adapt to yet more, "New Normals."

The Bible: Psalm 28:7

> "The Lord is my strength and my shield;
> My heart trusts in Him, and I am helped.
> My heart leaps for joy and I will
> Give thanks to Him…"

About "New Normals"

New Normals is a Nonprofit Corporation committed to providing informational resources that encourage survivors of stroke/brain injury. Our mission is to reach survivors in the earliest possible stages of their recovery.

To achieve our goals and provide the best sources of information we'd appreciate hearing from you. If you would like to participate we are currently looking for the following:

1. Your survivor stories of stroke/brain injury
2. Many survivors want to return to work. Any information regarding returning to work.
3. Did you use the government's "Ticket to Work" program through disability? Did you start your own business? Do you work from home?
4. Do you have "Best Practices" that aided in your recovery?
5. Your story of gratitude as it relates to the stroke/ brain injury.

Please provide contact information. Before we use your submission we will contact you.

You can send your stories to us-

Address: *New Normals Inc.*
           P.O. BOX 935
           Hanover, PA. 17331

Via email: Newnormals1@aol.com

OR visit our website: www.newnormals.com

*A percentage of profits from this book will be donated to support the advancement of Survivors of Stroke/Brain Injury.

LaVergne, TN USA
21 September 2009
158501LV00002B/89/P